EVERYDAY
HEALTH AND
FITNESS
WITH
MULTIPLE
SCLEROSIS

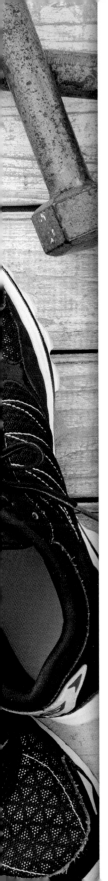
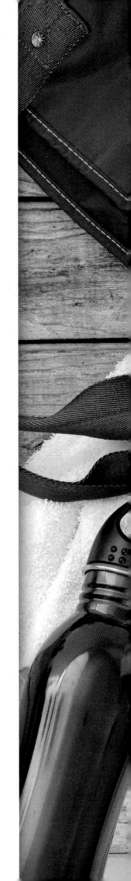

EVERYDAY
HEALTH AND
FITNESS
WITH
MULTIPLE
SCLEROSIS

· ·

Achieve Your Peak
Physical Wellness While
Working with Limited Mobility

· ·

DAVID LYONS

FOUNDER OF MS FITNESS CHALLENGE

WITH JACOB SLOANE, M.D., PH.D.

NEUROLOGIST AT BETH ISRAEL DEACONESS MEDICAL CENTER

FAIR WINDS

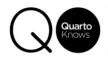

Quarto is the authority on a wide range of topics.

Quarto educates, entertains and enriches the lives of our readers—enthusiasts and lovers of hands-on living.

www.QuartoKnows.com

First published in the United States of America in 2017 by
Fair Winds Press, an imprint of
Quarto Publishing Group USA Inc.
100 Cummings Center, Suite 406-L
Beverly, Massachusetts 01915-6101
Telephone: (978) 282-9590
Fax: (978) 283-2742
QuartoKnows.com
Visit our blogs at QuartoKnows.com

21 20 19 18 17   1 2 3 4 5

ISBN: 978-1-59233-741-5

Digital edition published in 2017

Library of Congress Cataloging-in-Publication Data
Names: Lyons, David, 1958- author. | Sloane, Jacob, author.
Title: Everyday health and fitness with multiple sclerosis : achieve your peak physical wellness while working with limited mobility / David Lyons, Founder of MS Fitness Challenge, with Jacob Sloane, M.D., Neurologist, Beth Israel Deaconess Medical Center.
Description: Beverly, Massachusetts : Fair Winds Press, 2017. | Includes index.
Identifiers: LCCN 2016032289 | ISBN 9781592337415 (paperback)
Subjects: LCSH: Multiple sclerosis--Popular works. | Self-care, Health--Popular works. | BISAC: HEALTH & FITNESS / Diseases / Nervous System (incl. Brain). | HEALTH & FITNESS / Exercise. | HEALTH & FITNESS / Healthy Living.
Classification: LCC RC377 .L97 2017 | DDC 616.8/34--dc23
LC record available at https://lccn.loc.gov/2016032289

Cover Design: Laura Shaw Design, Inc., Lshawdesign.com
Cover Image: Glen Scott Photography
Design: Kathie Alexander
Photography: Robert Randall Productions, all exercise photos; Shutterstock, pages 27 (upper right), 56, 65; Daymond John, page 8; David Lyons, pages 27 (upper left and lower images), and 188 (upper image); courtesy Beth Israel Deaconess Medical Center, page 188, lower image.

Printed in China

The information in this book is for educational purposes only. It is not intended to replace the advice of a physician or medical practitioner. Please see your health care provider before beginning any new health program.

I cannot express enough the importance of the love and encouragement of my parents, Simon and Shirley, who taught me from childhood the meaning of hard work, dedication, and integrity, as they demonstrated all of those traits. They never looked at me as disabled when MS became part of my life, but, instead, told me this was an opportunity to demonstrate the ability to overcome any obstacle put in my path. I am honored to be their son. I pray that in my life's story, I come close to that as a role model to my children, Dean, Anna, Deric, Kalie, Christian, and Kara. I am proud of each of you.

And at the end of each day and the beginning of the next, I have been blessed with the most amazing, loving, and forgiving wife in Kendra, who has stood by my side through the difficulties MS has presented in our lives. She is amazing in her support of my goals no matter how difficult they are and despite the stress they impart. She is loving–in her immense heart for me and her patience of the bodybuilding lifestyle I have immersed her in. She is forgiving–in her unconditional, unwavering love through the roller coaster of physical symptoms and emotional tension MS brings into our lives. Kendra is the love of my life, and this life and this book, above all, are dedicated to her.

I have been blessed with a gracious God, in Jesus Christ, who has never let me down despite my shortcomings. It is His acceptance and love despite my imperfections, His mercy in my faults, and His grace undeserving that have given me the confidence to take on an incurable disease head on. And it is His strength in this battle that has empowered me from victory to victory.

2 TIMOTHY 4:17

CONTENTS

Foreword by Daymond John **8**

Introduction **9**

Part 1 — Preparing for Change and a Healthier You

1 Just Get Moving
Find Motivation and Inspiration **12**

2 Achieve Mental Fitness
Make Lifestyle Changes for a Healthy Mind **25**

3 Everyday Nutrition
Eat Right to Reach Your Goals **34**

Part 2 — The Multi-Phase Plan to Achieve Your Optimal Body

4 Getting Started
Know the Terms and Tools **54**

5 Phase 1
Adapt Your Workouts, Build Muscle, and Lose Fat **68**

6 Phase 2
Jump-Start Your Metabolism **121**

Acknowledgments **186**

About the Authors **188**

Appendix: Sample Fitness and Nutrition Journal **189**

Index **190**

FOREWORD by **Daymond John**, star of ABC's *Shark Tank*

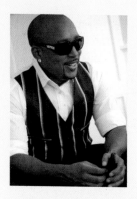

I have known David Lyons for some time now, and I have seen how much his motto–"never quit"–makes all the difference in his journey battling multiple sclerosis (MS).

I have been involved in the health and fitness industry, in one way or another, for many years. I have seen many fitness programs, fad diets, quick-results exercise regimens, and hundreds of ways the experts have hit the market with their systems. What I have never seen is a program, such as the OptimalBody HD Training System, the basis for *Everyday Health and Fitness with Multiple Sclerosis.*

I have personally worked with and consulted numerous individuals in the fitness industry who bring their methods to the marketplace, but the OptimalBody HD Training System is the first all-inclusive system for the millions of people who suffer through life with disabilities, challenges, and roadblocks to getting, and staying, in shape.

David has delivered an easy-to-follow program for this much-needed population. I cannot think of a better expert to bring this program to life than a man who lives these challenges every day. Despite his battle against MS, my friend David has beaten the odds and inspired millions of people worldwide with his resilience to prevent an incurable disease from controlling his life. He has worked with people across the globe–thanks to his charity, the MS Fitness Challenge–to help them achieve their fitness goals in spite of MS. Now, with this book, he is able to reach a multitude of people who want to get in and stay in shape by overcoming the obstacles they face.

It is likely that most of us will face our own trials in life that we need to push past. None of us is spared hardship and challenges. It's how we view these challenges that will either make us or break us. I wasn't always as successful as I am today. I worked hard, I endured hardship, and I fought my way here. I struggled through life's tests. I do not have a disease, as David does, nor do I have physical limitations, but I understand what it means to take a negative situation and turn it into a positive force in my life. This is exactly what David helps everyone do with the OptimalBody HD Training System. Through *Everyday Health and Fitness with Multiple Sclerosis*, he helps navigate you through the hard bumps and barriers that prevent many from succeeding in living their healthiest life.

> David's approach to life and fitness is an encouragement to all that there is hope and a plan to assist and support you toward the lifestyle you want.

David's approach to life and fitness is an encouragement to all that there is hope and a plan to assist and support you toward the lifestyle you want. You can have a new life of strength, empowerment, and control through David's philosophy and methodology. You now have a blueprint to follow as you take command of your body.

As I watched David receive the Health Advocate Lifetime Achievement Award from Arnold Schwarzenegger, the greatest bodybuilder of all time, I knew my friend had conquered what he was told would defeat him. And now, he will help you do the same. There are two words that come to mind when I think of David and the OptimalBody HD Training System: Never quit!

–Daymond John

There are many options to choose from when it comes to fitness programs that speak to the general population–people who want to get fit and transform their bodies. But where does that leave those of us challenged by an obstacle, such as a chronic disease, disability, or even a mental block or fear, but wanting to take the proper steps to live a healthy lifestyle?

The fitness market you see in infomercials and magazines sells beach bodies and ripped abs to people who are already in pretty good shape or are desparate for results, who will eagerly jump onto the next great workout craze. The rest of us, those facing real challenges and needing the most help and direction, are generally overlooked.

After being diagnosed with multiple sclerosis (MS), I knew I needed to come to grips with having an incurable disease that wanted to destroy my nervous system and defeat me. However, I was also determined not to let it beat me. I started to envision myself fighting against it. Because I couldn't find any fitness programs tailored to the specific needs of a person with multiple sclerosis, or any physical limitations for that matter, my training partner, Darren Barnes, and I decided to create that program. After seeing the extraordinary results from my own fitness journey, I decided it was time to share my philosophy with my community of peers, those of us with some form of disability that we need to conquer each day.

Everyday Health and Fitness with Multiple Sclerosis is a step-by-step instructional, educational, and comprehensive guide that, instead of setting unrealistic goals filled with hype, offers realistic advice to achieve a lifestyle of fitness and health despite your limitations.

This is not just a fitness book. In chapter 1 on motivation and inspiration, I share my personal journey before and after being diagnosed with MS, ranging from despair to achievement. Chapter 2 on mental fitness addresses how keeping your mind fresh, focused, and positive is as important as working your body. A fitness program is not only about how you exercise, but also what you fuel your body with every day, in and out of the gym. In chapter 3 on nutrition, registered dietitian Monica Pelle joins me to offer her expert advice on the foods and meal plans that bring optimal health and nutrition, especially when managing a chronic condition.

Throughout the book, you'll find expert advice by noted neurologist Jacob Sloane, M.D., Ph.D., who treats MS patients at the multiple sclerosis clinic at Beth Israel Deaconess Medical Center in Boston. Incorporating his Doctor's Notes, this book offers a medical perspective on the different symptoms and safety concerns associated with MS. Though we focus on MS, this program can be adapted to any condition or roadblock you may have.

Finally, *Everyday Health and Fitness with Multiple Sclerosis* introduces you to the foundation of fitness—the OptimalBody HD Training System—a program that trains the body as a whole and will help you attain your ultimate goal, no matter your current fitness level. The OptimalBody program was designed for all people with specific limitations. Those of us with disabilities, and those who may have other obstacles that limit them in one way or another, will all benefit from this program.

The terms *disability* and *limitation* imply that something cannot be done—but that's not true. Both Darren and I believe, and have proven, that through hard work and proper education, any goal can be attained. Sometimes the path to that goal has to be modified or altered, but, with perseverance, the goal can be accomplished.

Darren and I team up to take you through the phases of this system. It begins with a beginner stage (Phase 1) and advances to intermediate (Phase 2). We make it simple to adapt the training system to your needs and even make working out in a wheelchair possible and effective.

Strong minds and bodies are immensely powerful, and, regardless of our obstacles, we should always try to rise to meet them. It doesn't matter whether it's a simple fear of failure. If you can find the courage to fight for your goals, nothing can stop you.

We all go through struggles. When I go through my own personal struggles and my fight to beat MS, I think back to my father, Simon, a survivor of five Holocaust camps, who first instilled in me the beliefs that I still rely on today. For more than five years of his young life, he witnessed torture and death. Nonetheless, he never quit in his belief that he could get past these obstacles and survive, despite their severity. He is now ninety-three years old.

I also relate to my mother who, without a college education, rose to an executive position with American Express in a time when women did not have the opportunities they have today. These were obstacles she was able to overcome through a strong belief in herself and her own abilities.

And then there is my wife, Kendra, who continues to help others as she stands by me in this journey. No matter what is thrown in her path and no matter how many bad days I face with MS, she never quits breaking through the barriers life sets in her way. Therefore, all of us, in one way or another, face major obstacles in our lives. The key to overcome them is to be confident that there is a way to a better and healthier lifestyle. Let this book be your guide to better everyday health and fitness.

PREPARING
FOR
CHANGE
AND A
HEALTHIER
YOU

Just Get Moving
Find Motivation and Inspiration

People often ask when they begin an exercise program, "How can I get motivated?" It's a great question but, unfortunately, it doesn't have an easy answer.

Everyone has different physical and emotional needs and obstacles. We would all love to simply set a goal, work hard, and achieve it, but it's not that simple. Two important keys to success are inspiration and motivation. You have to find inspiration, dig deep inside yourself, locate that motivation, and keep a firm grip on it to strive toward and achieve your goals.

MY MOTIVATION

I have been lucky to find a lot of inspiration throughout my life from athletes, such as Muhammad Ali, and businessmen, such as Daymond John, who became successes despite their challenges. In general, I find it easy to stay motivated. But at the age of forty-seven, my foundation of motivation, achievement, and success was shaken. That was the year I was diagnosed with multiple sclerosis. After an attack by the disease that left me virtually paralyzed, I fought the depressing fact that I was no longer the same man I was before being diagnosed with this insidious disease. I spent most of my time visiting doctors, trying to manage what was happening to my body.

At night, I would lie awake trying to comprehend these new challenges and wondering how to cope. How was I going to fight the disease? In the past, I fought mental, emotional, and physical challenges by turning to fitness and amassing physical strength. But because of MS, I no longer had the physical capabilities to fight in the same way. MS had given me a noticeable limp, and I was now dragging my left leg as I walked. I was embarrassed to be seen in my condition, and I endured many sleepless nights.

While lying awake, I would contemplate my life with a new humility. I sought purpose and questioned everything. As a result, I was lost—floundering in an existence of self-pity and doubt that contradicted the foundational beliefs of my soul.

As a man of Christian faith, I have always believed that things happen for a reason, but I found myself doubting this was true. It was a pivotal new season of my life, and I realized it was time to reevaluate my purpose, goals, and direction. With what I know to be God's strength, I slowly emerged from my cocoon and began incorporating a few routine activities into my life again so I could establish a feeling of normalcy. It was time to get inspired!

Bodybuilding as Inspiration and Motivation

As a gym owner in my twenties and thirties, bodybuilding had been my sport of choice. In my forties, I ran a television production company and worked out in the gym routinely, but not as a competitive bodybuilder. When MS hit me, I knew I had to return to the gym and become whole again, but it took me a year before I returned. With the physical complications of MS, I had all but given up working out. So I started looking to bodybuilders who trained despite adversity. I knew it would be better to get away from distracting thoughts about my MS and focus on the fact that I was still alive.

My first goal in this positive line of thinking was to return to the gym. With impaired coordination, a dwindled body, and lingering numbness and pain, it was one of the most difficult things I've ever done. But I knew if I wanted to stay sane, I would have to push myself beyond my comfort level.

I had a membership to a health club minutes away from my home, so I began to plan a strategy. *How could I get to the gym and avoid being noticed by neighbors or embarrassed when strangers saw me holding onto machines to steady myself?* The gym was multi-leveled and expansive, which meant there were plenty of places to hide, and if I trained when it opened at 5:30 a.m., I'd likely have the place to myself. I started to think going unnoticed was possible. I found motivation through my faith and determination to change my life. I was not about to let MS dictate how I lived; I had to take control.

I was nervous, of course, but I pushed myself through the anxiety and stepped inside. My anxieties swam in my head: *Would I be able to do what I had planned? Would others see me as disabled? What if I couldn't stick with the training?* It truly took super-human motivation to push me forward and to be committed to my workout. Processing and coping with the emotions that arose when entering the gym and finishing the workout proved transformational.

I learned that the key to powerful motivation is looking at your alternatives and asking, "If I do this, where will I be?" and "What are the negative consequences if I *don't* follow through?" The power that came from blending positive personal motivation with the negative reality of defeat was that driving force that led me to accomplish my goal.

 Doctor's Note

Motivation is important, but so is your workout strategy. Patients should start exercising with a specific plan to avoid injury. Consider common MS symptoms, such as fatigue, weakness, balance, coordination, and heat intolerance, among others, before establishing an exercise plan.

Reclaiming My Life

That first day, I walked into the workout area wearing a headset blaring loud music. I was in my own world–my own zone. Much to my delight, there were fewer than ten people working out at that hour. They were spread out so far that I would have had to run into someone purposely to get their attention. I could stumble around and fall over, and no one would see or care. My prayers had been answered.

Strangely, though, even with my many years as a gym owner, boxer, and bodybuilder, I felt lost among the weights and machines. It had been more than a year since my diagnosis, and my body had grown accustomed to inactivity. I worked out slowly, using very light weights and doing small movements. I used weight-lifting straps to prevent dropping weights and injury. Because of my MS, it was difficult to maneuver around and get in and out of the equipment; I could barely hold onto the bars and weights with my left hand.

When I look back at this experience, and even as I deal with my MS symptoms today, the tingling and numbness did not cause much difficulty in my workouts. It was more the spasticity in movements, the shaking in my legs (especially my left one), and the fatigue that made working out such a chore.

The new safety challenges added difficulty to my exercise plans. To ensure I didn't injure myself, I took my time moving from one spot to another. I held onto equipment or braced myself against a wall to maintain balance. Before long, I didn't care what anyone thought or whether they were staring at me. The movements caused me pain and intensified the MS-induced tingling throughout my body, but I didn't care. I was working out!

Despite the fact that workouts heightened my MS symptoms, I continued to go to the gym four days a week. It just felt good to move and use my body again. Working out once more was one of the biggest steps I took to reclaim my life.

It wasn't long after that a close bodybuilder friend of mine, John, began talking to me about getting back into training. He knew I was going to the local gym because his wife worked out there. John also knew I was a hardcore bodybuilder most of my life through the many hours we spent exchanging training programs and nutritional regimens. He could tell I was hesitant about training because of my MS, but he thought it would be a great idea for me to go to a bodybuilding gym instead of a luxury fitness center.

John told me about his own workouts with his training partner, Darren Barnes, a certified fitness trainer, amateur competitive bodybuilder, and manager of a bodybuilding gym. I realized how much I missed that kind of training and how much I hated not being as big and strong as I had been before MS. I wanted to travel back to the 1980s—a time when I owned gyms and lived for bodybuilding—but here I was, almost forty-nine, and suffering from an incurable neurological disease.

John didn't want to hear my excuses. Except for safety issues, he couldn't see anything holding me back. He kept hinting that I should go to his gym and work out with him and Darren, but I thought he was crazy. How could I train with guys like them and keep up? I got embarrassed just thinking about going to a gym filled with bodybuilders. I didn't want them to see me having trouble moving around and struggling just to lift light weights. I may have been motivated, but not enough to step even further out of my comfort zone.

Facing My Fears

One day John showed up at my door, ready to go to the gym to train with Darren. He told me to put on my workout clothes and get in his car. I didn't want to do what he asked, but John was a big, powerful guy—a strong-willed Florida state trooper, as a matter of fact. If he'd wanted to, he could have picked me up, thrown me into his car, and forced me to go. But his presence was what I needed to act on my motivation.

Though hard to admit, I was deeply grateful that John took action, even if I was scared. In fact, just before John showed up that day, I had been building my confidence and telling myself I could be a person without a disability once again. I had been finding greater motivation to take my body to the next level; I was just struggling to get there. It's the mental battle we all face when trying to manifest the confidence we need to move ahead.

When we arrived at the gym, Darren was waiting for us. John and Darren first addressed our top priority—safety. They knew about my spasticity and other symptoms and made a plan to be by my side at all times to ensure I did not hurt myself. They set up benches and weights for each exercise and were ready to help me coordinate and control every aspect of each one.

Now after years of being a leader in the gym, I had to follow the lead of my training partners. Darren and John were extremely patient and helpful in getting me through my workout without easing up prematurely. As we worked out, I found that fatigue was the most daunting challenge. I tried to keep up the pace, but it was evident I was struggling. Increasing fatigue during lifting sessions made it hard for me to judge how much to lift and how to maximize safety.

The guys witnessed my coordination problems and inability to grasp the weights securely for upper chest and triceps workouts. It had been such a long time since I'd pushed myself to that level, and I felt the pain and other symptoms of MS. But after coming that far, there wasn't any way I was going to stop training that day. John and Darren stood by me and encouraged me despite this obstacle.

I was blessed. I had supportive friends to help push me. But with or without them, I was the one who had to do the training. Ultimately, the motivation and drive to do this had to come from within. It was a great lesson: You have to find a way to take charge of your own motivation with or without the help of others. If certain family members or friends see your vision, get them on board, even if, just as cheerleaders. And if you don't have anyone who will work out with you, the gym itself can be a great resource. Just as I found Darren, stay alert for someone at the gym looking, as you are, for a workout partner. Although a personal trainer can provide the ultimate in encouragement, not everybody can afford one. But remember, whether you find that fitness buddy or can afford a trainer, you can uncover that inner strength on your own. You are the one who ultimately determines your destiny, and this book can be your workout buddy along the way.

When we finished the workout that day, the sense of accomplishment I felt was astounding. There was no doubt in my mind that I would become a bodybuilder again, regardless of the level of intensity I could handle. It was clear to me that, when it comes to our minds, we are alone. Nobody can make the decision for us to achieve higher goals. And through that experience in the gym, my mind started believing positive truths about my ability and countering the negative, self-defeating thoughts. That workout proved to me I had the strength in mind and body to push myself through the adversity of MS step by step.

One Workout at a Time

Step by step meant one workout at a time. John and Darren agreed I could keep training with them, and John gave me a weekly workout schedule. He picked me up each training day,

 Doctor's Note

Fatigue is an important and common issue for those with MS. People with MS should be aware of how they feel and mindful of their energy levels before exercising. Also, fatigue may worsen with exercise, so it is important to listen to your body and stop if needed.

and we'd ride together to the gym. I had a routine, a schedule, and a plan—important keys to staying on track to a goal.

I soon discovered, though, that just because you start the task, it doesn't necessarily get easier. I may have been on my way and training as a bodybuilder again, but that didn't make the symptoms of MS miraculously disappear. I still battled them daily, with each new sunrise bringing uncertain challenges. The symptoms, ranging from numbness to spasticity to fatigue, existed with or without the workouts. I was tired when I woke up, tired when I worked out, and tired when I went to bed. There wasn't a time I wasn't tired. But I could either be tired and be a bodybuilder again, or I could be tired and let my body deteriorate.

Life is not a straight path. Even when we're motivated, we all face ups, downs, victories, and setbacks. Things weren't any easier on my forty-ninth birthday than they were when I was first diagnosed at forty-seven. Every time I looked to the side using my left eye, all I could see was darkness, as if a black hole had taken over my vision.

My thoughts were often a cloud of lost names and sentences without words. I struggled to find traces of thoughts I'd once been able to reach without effort. My body was unrecognizable to me, and I was nothing like the man I'd been less than two years ago. I contemplated my life and found it hard to accept this was it–that this was me. After almost a half century of hard work, I felt defeated. My birthday celebrated a life that had been torn from me in many ways.

I often closed my eyes and prayed that everything I'd once had would reappear and that it had all been just a terrible nightmare. I wanted to open my eyes and have my health and my body be whole again, but this was no nightmare. I was in a body that no longer cooperated with a mind that found it hard to grasp simple thoughts. I constantly asked, "Now what?"

At forty-nine, the reflection staring back at me in the mirror seemed foreign. It wasn't me. It was a man with an incurable disease struggling to complete light workouts at the gym. *What had happened to the Dave who'd had endless energy? Where was the guy who pushed himself in the gym to the point of bending bars?* That twenty-year-old athlete was in there somewhere; I just knew it. I had to find something to save my body as it tried to destroy itself. I had to reach back to find that powerful version of me.

This challenge to my motivation proved beneficial. It was like a muscle workout but for my emotions. Although, my motivation was torn down, it began to take stronger root–as a tree must be pruned for it to grow healthy and strong.

As I began to accept reality, my desire to beat the odds grew. I had a choice. I could put on my armor, grab my weapon, and fight the battle like the warrior I claimed to be, or I could lay down my weapons and let the disease ravage me. I chose to fight. And I found that the power came from within as I battled the enemy. That day–December 10, 2007–I resolved to undertake a challenge that would push my mind, body, and spirit to their limits. It marked the beginning of my personal journey to a place few had ventured and led me to accomplish what no one my age with MS had ever achieved.

When we look at where we are in our lives, when we examine our circumstances and physical state, when we recognize what it is we want to accomplish, only then can we put a plan in motion to get there. At this point, we find the motivation to reach our goals.

I want to challenge you, despite your obstacles, physical limitations, and adversities, to look at yourself as a warrior ready to go into battle. Visualize yourself defeating the enemy, regardless of what that enemy is. See yourself in the gym or at home training to the highest level. Now look in the mirror, see yourself for who you are, and ask, "Am I inspired? Am I motivated to succeed?" I hope this book will help motivate you for this task. You will get there, just like I did.

MY MS BODYBUILDING CHALLENGE

My personal journey began when I made the decision to stand against the disease and create my own MS bodybuilding challenge. From that day, my life would take a different path. In my mind, I wasn't an MS patient anymore. I was a man who had to beat the odds and overcome this disease.

That day, I decided to take on the incredible, odds-defying challenge of competing in a high-level, amateur bodybuilding contest at the age of fifty. No one with MS had ever done that. And I also intended to forego the division of people with disabilities and enter as a regular contestant. I was determined to stand on stage next to the healthy athletes and compete against them with no special considerations.

I hadn't stepped onto a bodybuildoing contest stage in more than twenty-five years, and I hadn't trained competitively for at least fifteen years (long before I was diagnosed). Even if I was healthy, I wouldn't be anywhere near the condition of today's amateur National Physique Committee (NPC) bodybuilders. With the advancements in diet and training, and the abundance of performance-enhancing drugs and supplements, amateur bodybuilding had been taken to a new level that far surpassed the pros of my day. But to me it wasn't about winning. It was a personal challenge not to give up on life.

That day, I told John about my plan. He wasn't as shocked as I thought he'd be, and he responded, "If anyone can do this, you can." I didn't tell Darren until after the workout that day. To do this successfully, I would need a trainer who could develop a specific bodybuilding routine and diet for me, and I wanted him to be the one. It just seemed natural for me to ask Darren; he had been training with me for awhile and knew what I went through during each session. Plus, he was a certified fitness trainer working with winning amateur competitive bodybuilders, a top three-ranked competitive bodybuilder himself, and also an all-around great guy.

I explained to Darren the entire plan and philosophy for my MS bodybuilding challenge and expressed my passion to do it. His response was a little different than John's. "This is crazy," he said. "Are you sure you want to do this?" But after further thought, he agreed. "I'm in. I'll work on a diet and training routine. When do you want to start?"

I smiled. "Tomorrow."

This was a massive undertaking for Darren, and there had to be a starting point with a slow progression to my (truly, our) goal. During the first month or two, we worked on establishing a foundation of training that would prepare my body for much more grueling workouts. I also started maintaining a strict diet to put on much-needed muscle. John would continue training with us, but our focus would shift to getting me ready to compete. Darren was currently competing, so he was already in that groove. Between his guidance, John's encouragement, and my desire, I had the perfect combination of knowledge and motivation behind me.

As soon as we started, the training days began to peel away from the calendar, and I became increasingly more inspired. I knew in my heart there was a greater purpose in all of this. The disease, the refusal to give up on life and, now, my goal to complete an odds-defying task were, I believed, a bigger vision with a broader perspective.

One thing that drove me was knowing that by standing on a bodybuilding stage with MS, I would be able to affect others. I could be an example of how faith, strength, and willpower could move mountains—or simply rebuild muscles—in the face of disease. The excitement of moving my life forward in one area soon spilled over into others, and I knew it was a new chapter—one filled with hope and the belief that all things were possible.

As I mentioned, I am a man of faith. During this time, I relied on the Bible to supply me with courage and strength. I read the Scriptures and was particularly inspired by the account of Job—a man afflicted by major disease and stripped of everything he had; yet he persevered. To me, if Job could overcome those overwhelming afflictions and trials and remain strong in his faith, I could overcome living with MS and start life over at almost fifty years old. I stayed faithful to the training plan and diet and gained strength with each new day.

As the challenge progressed, we were also blessed with the help and support of a sports medicine doctor and a nutritional supplement company. The doctor donated his time to treat me, and the supplement company provided bodybuilding products as a sponsor of my purpose.

The cause gained momentum, and I decided to spread the word to the bodybuilding and fitness world. It was my deepest desire to show that through faith and motivation, anyone could overcome whatever odds stood against them. There was no reason someone shouldn't be able to achieve her goals and stay focused on a fitness program for life, which is why we eventually developed the OptimalBody HD Training System—to keep men and women on track with their fitness goals. (For more on the OptimalBody HD Training System, see chapter 4.) But this type of commitment wouldn't come without bumps in the road.

Feeling the Pressure

As the MS Bodybuilding Challenge wore on, I began to feel the pressure. I started to doubt whether I could handle the enormity of it all. *Could I really compete in a bodybuilding contest while having MS and stand up against healthy bodybuilders? Could I even walk onto the stage? Could I pose without losing my balance? Could I build any real muscle while my body was deteriorating from MS?* The questions, doubts, and uncertainties accumulated and threatened to pull me down. It was imperative to shut out negative thinking and stay focused on the goal.

Staying Focused

Darren's regimen was grueling. He pushed me to lift harder and be better each day—and slowly but surely I responded. With a solid training base, I entered a National Physique Committee (NPC) contest because of its high level of competition and to earn the respect of the bodybuilding community.

Darren questioned my taking on an NPC show. The athletes who competed in these contests were huge, ripped, and, often, performance-enhancing drug users, but I was determined to stand on an NPC stage regardless of the odds. After evaluating our options, we set our sights on Orlando's NPC Mid-Florida Classic bodybuilding contest in June 2009. With our goal in place, Darren and I went full-steam ahead. I told him to treat me as if I was any other client getting ready to compete. His focus was to put as much size on me as possible and push me to lift as much weight as I could.

I struggled, having little to no coordination. I was constantly fatigued, and I battled perpetual pain and numbness. It was extremely hard to grasp dumbbells and weight bars because I had trouble with my grip, especially in my left hand. I wrapped straps around my wrists and the weights to keep them in place when my fingers gave out and I lost all feeling. Often

Doctor's Note

Because of potential health risks, MS patients should exercise with trainers. Without direct supervision, patients may be at risk for injury.

when it came to the last reps of the final sets, the weights would actually be held by the straps instead of my fingers.

Another problem was the stiffness and numbness in my left arm and hand. If you'd stuck a knife in either one, I wouldn't have felt it. Although I could feel 90 percent of my right side, I could only feel 20 percent of my left. It had been that way ever since my major MS attack in 2006. Still, even though I had little feeling when it came to touch, I experienced tremendous pain from the MS symptoms.

Though MS is a complicated disease to understand, its symptoms are even more difficult to explain. There was a persistent sensation in my body similar to the pins-and-needles feeling of your arm or leg falling asleep. I was numb to the touch but endured painful tingling inside.

With the physical limitations of my left side, my left leg became the most problematic in terms of training. Not only did it have the awful pins and needles, but it also highlighted the nightmarish disconnect in my brain. Though I tried my hardest to coordinate that leg, it would still drag regardless of my efforts. I couldn't lift it the same way as I could my right, and performing leg movements during workouts was like trying to sprint when all you can do is walk.

Darren helped me get up from the leg press machine, and he helped me stay coordinated, holding onto my waist to stabilize my body during squats, because my left side was so numb. He also pulled up on my left leg when it lagged in leg extensions or curls. During every workout–upper and lower body–both of my legs would shake, the left one considerably more than the right one. And when I overheated, my skin would itch everywhere. With so many symptoms and side effects, it's challenging just to stay sane.

Within a short period of time, my five-foot-ten (1.75 m) body had gone from 165 lb (75 kg) of deteriorated flesh to 195 lb (88.5 kg) of muscle and bulk. The nutritional supplements, protein powder, and six meals a day, when combined with the training, were working. From the start, Darren had impressed me as someone who followed through and knew how to accomplish his goals, and he was certainly doing his job with me. He was a martial arts champion, as well as an amateur bodybuilding titleholder–and his drive was as intense as mine. We made a great team.

As the training results started to appear, I received more attention from the public. I'd been interviewed and featured in the media and was being sponsored by several major players in the industry. It was all a huge blessing, and I really was excited, but I also started to feel the pressure. With so many eyes on me, I wanted to train like a madman. If I was going to achieve the goal, I needed to train as hard as I'd done in my twenties, even if my body was vastly different. Much to my own displeasure, those differences made things a lot more challenging than I could have anticipated.

Ask any MS patient to name the one most persistent symptom of the disease, and he or she will probably say fatigue. We are constantly tired, and we need more rest than healthy people. Every day I struggled to get out of bed, and I had to dig deep to make it into the gym. On many occasions, that struggle proved to be a test of my faith more than my strength. I prayed for strength of body, mind, and spirit, and I chose to believe that God would give me the ability to face the day.

Building My Mental Muscles

Every time I trained, my symptoms would worsen and then take hours to subside. With the nerve damage I'd sustained from my initial MS attack, it was obvious that no matter how strong-willed I was, the symptoms weren't going to subside. No matter how hard my mind tried to convince me I was still the young, healthy bodybuilder who could bend bars in the gym, my body said something else. To keep moving forward, I had to recondition my thoughts to believe I actually *could* do whatever was set before me. That mental battle was every bit as exhausting as the physical one. It was a constant internal wrestling match. On some days, I was completely focused on the victory, while on others I questioned my choices.

I learned that thoughts snowball in whatever direction we allow them to go. When I entertained negative, self-doubting thoughts, more would surface regarding my ability to complete the challenge. Then if I let those thoughts take root, they would grow into doubts about my ability to train. If I let it get that far, it was tough to regain my composure.

The Path Is Never Straight

With the challenges of my symptoms and the daily mental battle, there were also other setbacks that threatened the challenge along the way. One of these stemmed from the fact that, due to my MS, I was now more susceptible to injuries. I was aware of the condition, so I knew I had to train hard but work smart and avoid lifting more than my body could handle. But just like any hardheaded bodybuilder, I didn't always do the wise thing. In my competitive bodybuilding days, I had been used to training six days a week for hours on end, but since that time studies have shown that more time is needed between sessions to achieve maximum muscle growth. Based on the competitors' performances who followed that philosophy, it appeared the studies were right.

For an old-school bodybuilder, though, the concept was difficult to believe. Darren wanted me to train four days a week with lighter weights, more repetitions, and slower movements;

I wanted to push heavy weights for fewer reps and use bursts of power. This was *not* the smart way to work out with MS, and I advise you never to follow this style of workout if you have MS, or any type of limiting condition.

On the days Darren wasn't with me, I snuck in my old training methods. Needless to say, he wasn't happy about it. He kept reminding me that as an MS-stricken fifty-year-old, I was more susceptible to injuries and that the last thing we needed was a torn muscle. "One injury could put an end to the MS bodybuilding challenge altogether," he'd say.

One late spring day in 2008, I learned my lesson the hard way. While training my own way and ignoring Darren's plan and advice, I tore my right pec lifting 400 lb (181 kg) on the bench press. I wasn't ready to face that I needed to train differently with MS. *There is absolutely no need to lift heavy weights for low repetitions under any circumstance when dealing with this disease.* In fact, unless you are training for power lifting, even healthy people do not need heavy weight lifting to become physically fit and in top shape. You will find this out while using the OptimalBody HD Training System.

I never attempt these ego lifts any more. I'd tried to prove something to my pride, and I wound up paying the price by suffering what my doctor said was the worst muscle tear

he'd ever seen. It took an entire six months to recover, and it derailed our first competition. Immediately after the injury, I sat on my couch with ice on my chest berating myself for likely ending the MS bodybuilding challenge—all because I was foolish. I was afraid to call Darren and tell him the news because it would be a slap in the face to his work. I had let him down and let myself down, too.

Darren was frustrated that all our hard work wouldn't get us to the June 2009 NPC contest, but he was more upset that I thought lifting heavy weights would get me to my goal faster. I had been impatient, looking for a shortcut. Shortcuts, though, are rarely a good way to make progress. I learned that transforming your body is a slow, methodical process. It requires patience, discipline, and strategy. There are no easy or fast-track ways to succeed long term, which is why so many fad diets and workouts cause people to remain on the fitness yo-yo for years. Through my injury, I learned a challenging lesson that eventually helped us create the Optimal-Body HD Training System.

Once I realized how important it was to follow wisdom and not forcefully rush the process, I was able to help our team develop a sustainable, viable plan that would allow others to achieve their physical goals, as well. Because, if it's one thing the world needs to hear, it's that those 30-day fitness blitzes that claim to change your body from flab to fit are nothing but hype. They can have short-term results but lead to long-term failures.

After my injury, Darren and I agreed we'd come too far to quit, and I realized I was more motivated than ever to succeed. Darren's positive attitude kept me from giving up.

Coming back from the injury was brutal. The tear had been so severe that I shocked my doctor the first few times I went in. Starting at the midpoint of my right pec, I was black, blue, and red down my right side and my right arm. During my first follow-up appointment, it was still too swollen to tell how much of the pec was torn, and whether it was torn with or without the tendon. If the tendon was torn along with the muscle, the doctor could repair it by stretching the tendon back with the muscle and reattaching it to the bone. However, if the tear was only muscle, the chances of repair were slight.

While we waited for the swelling to go down, I did what I could to salvage my training by working on my lower body. Three weeks after the incident, I went back to my doctor, and he examined the pec muscle. The exam results showed that it was, indeed, a muscle-only tear and not a tendon issue. After an MRI, it was discovered that I'd almost torn the muscle completely off the bone. It was ripped halfway into the center of my body, which had left me with a balled-up half of a right chest. The doctor said I was to take the recovery slowly and start training lightly in about five months.

To be honest, I only sort of followed his advice. This was a mistake. I wasn't willing just to sit around for five months when only one part of my body was injured. So, I went back into the gym the next Monday morning with a plan and a resolve not to be reckless. I am not suggesting you dismiss your doctor's advice, especially when I just advocated for following a strategic plan and being patient. I still had to be patient in the recovery and work on making smarter choices in my revised strategy. What I am saying, though, is that it's okay to fight for your mental and physical progress. You will

 Doctor's Notes

- Exercise can cause injuries more readily in people with MS. Weak bones from MS treatments, such as corticosteroids, can lead to arthritis or fractures. Muscle tears and trauma can occur, but they are most often manageable with massage, hot baths, and non-steroidal anti-inflammatories (NSAIDS), such as ibuprofen or prescription medicines.

  Injuries can result from MS symptoms, as well. So, take care in exercising weak regions of the body because it is difficult to know how these regions will behave during exercise, both over the short and long term. Use weight-lifting straps and other accommodations if there are safety risks, which can be assessed by professional trainers and therapists.

  Fatigue and heat intolerance in people with MS can lead to injury because fatigue can make you less attentive. Heat can worsen symptoms of weakness, numbness, or incoordination during exercise. Muscles can progressively fatigue so pay close attention to changes in your body while you exercise.

- Sustained exercise and diet plans, as opposed to quick-fix solutions, lead to sustained benefits.

have setbacks, but they are part of the process. Use your wisdom and stick to your plan, knowing you may have to work through some rough patches.

EYES ON THE PRIZE

Finally, in August 2009, I achieved my goal. Despite MS, age, and injury, I stood on the stage of the Florida State Bodybuilding Championship and competed against healthy bodybuilders of my class. No, I did not place. With a still-deformed right pec and a smaller frame than the other competitors, it was a victory that I made it there at all.

For my determination, though, I was awarded the most inspirational bodybuilder trophy by the event's organizers. Though that meant so much to me, the real payoffs were overcoming the obstacles, reclaiming my life, and inspiring others to believe they could do the same. It is my story, and stories like these, that can motivate others.

It's not the win or the loss that matters; it's the journey to the goal and dream that makes you victorious. Not everyone will achieve the same results from the same attempts, but if you are motivated to reach a desired outcome, all is possible.

I am certain you're thinking, "Everyone says to get motivated, and every trainer has a secret that will get you in shape in thirty days. So what's new with this program?" First, it's not a program; it's a lifestyle. I can tell you without hesitation that fitness is not a get-results-quick scheme, a miracle pill, or a stop-and-go rollercoaster. Fitness is a way of living. Once you grasp that notion, you will look at getting in the best shape of your life as simply the way you operate. Second, to keep your journey moving forward in spite of obstacles, though, you need to be inspired to be motivated. Whether it's through my story or someone else's, find your motivation and let it take you where you never thought possible. And read on to learn how to use the OptimalBody HD Training System on your road to fitness.

Doctor's Notes

- Doctors really try to give you the best advice they have to offer, so follow their advice. If they do not know something, they can refer you to specialists who do.

- Keep your doctor in the loop in terms of your exercise, whether you feel like it has been a good or bad effort, and whether it adhered to a set plan or deviated from it.

- David adapted his routine for specific problems he had. This is precisely what people with MS should do, whether symptoms are consistently present or fluctuate during exercise sessions.

Doctor's Note

Many MS patients are eager to begin exercising but lose interest soon after. Data indicates that most MS patients can steadily increase fitness with consistent long-term exercise. They can even recover function with consistent effort.

CHAPTER 2

Achieve Mental Fitness
Make Lifestyle Changes for a Healthy Mind

"You have the power to do anything you set your mind to." We have all been told this at some point in our lives, likely starting in childhood. The older we get, though, the more the power of these words begins to fade. With this book–and this chapter specifically–I aim to keep these words first and foremost in your mind!

My daughter Kara is a life coach, and she constantly reminds her clients about the importance of training our minds to improve our health, following a fitness and nutrition regimen, and staying the course in maintaining a lifestyle of health and fitness. In essence, a life coach is there to guide and cheer you on along the journey. You hold all the answers you need. The same applies to my role as your instructor through this book. As your fitness coach, I hope to guide and support you to a new lifestyle.

The mind can be a powerful tool when beginning a new fitness routine because that which consumes our mind will steer the direction we take in life. Marcus Aurelius once said, "You have power over your mind, not outside events. Realize this, and you will find strength." I believe these powerful words will resonate with most of you, especially as you change your daily routine from your norm, to one directed toward overcoming your boundaries and challenges.

Being diagnosed with MS was not my plan, nor did I expect to become a spokesperson for living with MS. But I focused my mind and made the conscious decision to become physically and mentally fit despite the roadblocks ahead. That mind-set placed me on the path I walk today. When it comes to our physical bodies and how we wish to use them or prefer them to look, gaining and maintaining firm control of our thoughts will allow us greater control over our bodies and the progress we seek to attain.

Controlling something as powerful as the mind takes time, effort, and dedication. Can I do it for you? Unfortunately not. The power is completely in you, and the beauty is, if you are ready and you want it, you are already fueled to move ahead!

> Controlling something as powerful as the mind takes time, effort, and dedication.

MEDITATION

We have all heard of meditation, and many of us have even tried it in some form. Though meditation has long been a therapeutic practice, it is more recently recognized from a scientific perspective for its health benefits. Studies have shown that meditation increases mental strength, focus, memory retention, and recall. It enhances cognitive skills, creative thinking, problem solving, and decision-making.

Meditation also contributes to higher information processing by enhancing the ability to ignore distractions. Moreover, it has been shown to boost the immune system and energy levels and improve breathing, heart rate, and blood pressure, as well as help reduce heart issues, brain problems, and inflammatory disorders—all the while contributing to greater longevity.

It can feel unfamiliar, even strange, to sit in silence and be alone with your thoughts in this fast-paced world. There is no need to master meditation immediately, but the benefits come fast. Meditation can, in short duration, bring you peace, comfort, simplicity, stillness, motivation, joy, and love. It may help you focus on your exercise and nutritional plans, so you can follow through to your goals.

Doctor's Note

Multiple studies show that meditation reduces the risk of depression, anxiety, and fatigue and increases quality of life. With MS, evidence suggests that meditation also leads to higher cognitive function as assessed by meditating patients. This is largely due to patients exploring thoughts and emotions instead of reacting to them. Unfortunately, there is no evidence that meditation alters the disease course, including relapses or progressive symptoms. It does make sense, however, that meditation can reduce stress that could contribute to relapse risk. In addition, meditation can clearly help manage ongoing symptoms, including depression, anxiety, and fatigue.

Kara suggests the following steps to many clients. If you feel you cannot complete a step or that it is too hard, Kara will tell you, "You need it more than ever, then!" Once again, this is a practice. It can be intimidating or overwhelming but as I have followed my daughter's advice, it has helped my mental fitness tremendously.

Here are a few simple tips to start meditating:

- **Begin slowly.** Set a timer for five minutes and increase by one minute each time you meditate. Try for thirty or more minutes a day but don't overwhelm yourself. Instead, enjoy the process.

- **Keep an elevated posture.** If this hurts too much, then make yourself comfortable. However, when you hold an elevated posture, you feel more open to your body's circulation.

- **Notice your breathing.** The pace of breathing is so important during meditation. Maintain focus as you slowly breathe in and then out.

- **Create an appropriate mood.** Light candles, spray your favorite scent, and release yourself from distractions.

- **Stay with your practice.** Once you begin experiencing the benefits of meditation, it is probable you will add it to your daily routine. Stay encouraged.

- **Trust your feelings.** You can meditate in silence, to relaxing music, or whatever you feel is best for you.

YOGA

Yoga is thought to have originated in India five thousand years ago but may be traced back even further than that. How beautiful is the opportunity to enjoy such an ancient practice that so many before us have taken part in? It is no wonder yoga has remained in our cultures for so long. Its benefits are genuinely remarkable. Yoga helps your body and strengthens your mind, as well. Concentration and focus are key; you must clear your mind of all distractions. Yoga incorporates breathing techniques, as well as meditation. In fact, yoga is said to have been created to help individuals meditate longer and strengthen the body to allow them to remain sitting for a longer period of time. Simply, yoga is amazing for your body. More than that, it brings balance to life, which is important to mental fitness. Reducing stress through yoga is especially crucial for people with MS. I cannot tell you how many times, while participating in a sweaty, focused yoga class, I have experienced a tremendous release of stress.

Yoga classes are everywhere these days. You can even find free online classes (Doyogawithme.com has free yoga classes any time, any day). You can find a range of yoga types based on your personal goals, preferred style, and fitness level. If you haven't tried it yet, give it a shot.

POSITIVE AFFIRMATIONS

As a man of faith, my Bible tells me that we reap what we speak or believe. So, whether or not you look at this concept in a spititual way, it means we can become what we desire and achieve what we imagine. Now is your chance to start a simple practice every day to recognize the small, important things in life while remaining focused on the positive and your

 Doctor's Note

Research shows that yoga helps reduce pain and fatigue, while increasing quality of life for prople with MS. Functional strength and balance can respond to yoga, as well. Certain yoga approaches can even help with urinary symptoms in MS.

goals. Saying (or thinking) affirmations to yourself daily helps you maintain a constant state of gratitude.

This practice also helps you become more aware of your daily thoughts, even if this is new for you. If you are aware and open to a fresh way of thinking, possibilities that were previously closed to you will begin to open. I have worked with and spoken to many people who wanted to change their fitness lifestyle, and the first step is always to change their mental fitness. It's too easy to focus on pain, defeat, obstacles, and other negative thoughts. But once you are able to maintain a positive, affirmative attitude, you can ignite success.

A wonderful thing about positive affirmations is that you can create anything your mind is as capable, creative, or detailed as you choose. Start with a simple affirmation, such as:

- Today I am thankful I can exercise.
- I am going to have a great workout today. I am here for a reason, and I am going to conquer my goals.
- Congratulations! I did not eat that cookie!

Communicate positive things to yourself and express gratitude for who you are despite your challenge. Don't let your condition, disability, or obstacle determine who you are and what you believe in. Once you begin this sort of self-communication, you start to believe it, you begin to live it, and you become it.

Place sticky notes around the house with positive statements or inspiration quotations that you say or read every day. Leave others for your spouse, friends, or colleagues. I remind myself that MS is a disease that I have, not a disease that controls me. Every day, I affirm that I can conquer MS, I can break through obstacles, and I can succeed in my goals to create a better body in spite of what looks impossible to others. More importantly, I work to become a better me in all I am and to help others become better, as well.

If you have trouble coming up with affirmations, look some up to help get started. One such resource is *The Affirmation Spot* (theaffirmationspot.wordpress.com/2012/01/09/41-health-fitness-and-weight-loss-affirmations), which offers sixty-four affirmations for health, fitness, and weight loss. *Affirm Your Life* is another great blog that will inspire you with a variety of affirmations on fitness (affirmyourlife.blogspot.com/2009/07/fitness-affirmations.html).

If you don't find the affirmation that fits you or your goals, it's easy to convert one to a personal vision. For example, I converted the affirmation "Step by step and rep by rep, I am creating my perfect body" to "Step by step and rep by rep, I am beating MS in the gym." Just as with anything, with practice comes habit, and with habit comes permanent change. Eventually, they will roll right off your tongue, onto a sticky note, or through your mind, especially once you experience the benefits.

VISION BOARD

A vision board is a tool used to help clarify, concentrate, and maintain focus on your life goals. It may be a physical board or a virtual one (such as a Pinterest board) on which you display images and words that represent whatever you want to be, do, or have in your life. In this case, you should collect images or items that represent a lifestyle of fitness, nutrition, and health for you–not just what someone tells you it is. Creating a vision board allows you to visualize positive affirmations more clearly.

Vision boards have proven to offer measurable results in my personal life. They are one of the most effective tools for instilling and maintaining a positive attitude, and visualization is a truly powerful exercise. *Psychology Today* reports that the brain patterns activated when a weightlifter lifts heavy weights are also similarly activated when the lifter simply imagines (visualizes) lifting weights.

Many famous and accomplished athletes use vision boards as a functional tool, such as Arnold Schwarzenegger, Olympic gold medalist skier Lindsey Vonn, and Kerri Walsh and Misty May-Treanor, the most successful female beach volleyball team in history. Consider using a vision board for getting you on the right track for your fitness and nutritional program.

Vision boards are a fun, creative outlet, as well as a great brain exercise. Not only should you post pictures of things you desire, but also photos of how you wish to feel or look. Cut pictures from magazines or print them from the Internet to post on the board. You can even put other things on the board that represent your goals. For example, on my new vision board, I fastened my competitor's number from my win of the 2009 Most Inspirational Bodybuilder trophy.

Another option is an online vision board using a collage application or Pinterest, which you can access on your computer, phone, or tablet. You can add, erase, or edit things at any time and it is super easy. You might use your vision board as a screen-saver so you are sure to look at it every day.

Make a board, place it where you will see it every day, engage with it, and absorb it. Feel the varying emotions your vision board stirs in you. When I look at my board with that number hanging on it, I feel like Rocky getting into the ring to fight Apollo Creed for the second time: I am pumped! That emotion helped me get my body to a level where it had not been since my twenties. I became leaner and more muscular than anyone thought I could at fifty-six years old with MS. To be honest, I even shocked myself when I looked at the pictures of me standing next to Arnold Schwarzanegger. For those of us who think visually or are motivated by results we can see or feel, vision boards can serve as a powerful tool.

Allow me to share a quick story about a holistic healer my daughter Kara visited in Sedona, Arizona. When she entered her office, Kara noticed a massive vision board on the healer's desk. At the end of the session, Kara asked her about it, and the healer explained that her vision board represents her

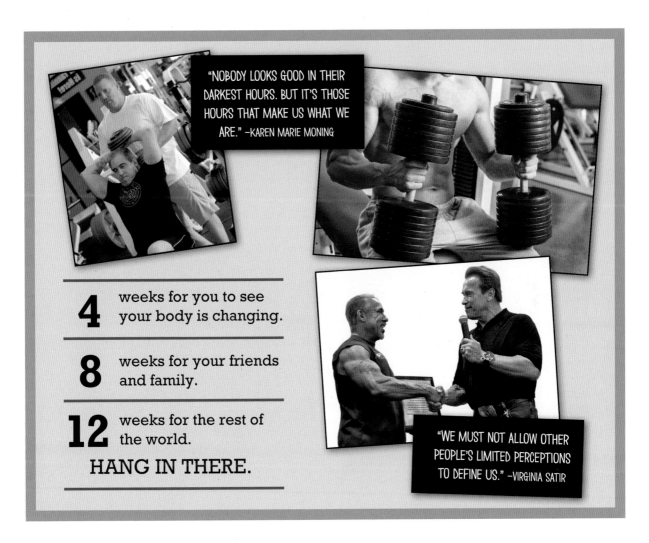

"NOBODY LOOKS GOOD IN THEIR DARKEST HOURS. BUT IT'S THOSE HOURS THAT MAKE US WHAT WE ARE." –KAREN MARIE MONING

4 weeks for you to see your body is changing.

8 weeks for your friends and family.

12 weeks for the rest of the world.

HANG IN THERE.

"WE MUST NOT ALLOW OTHER PEOPLE'S LIMITED PERCEPTIONS TO DEFINE US." –VIRGINIA SATIR

desires and challenges; one of those challenges occurred when doctors told her she would be unable to have children. She spent a lot of money on infertility treatments, but they did not work. Rather than give up, the healer created a vision board. She also practiced meditation, yoga, positive affirmations, acupuncture, and other holistic approaches to promote a healthy lifestyle and overcome her challenges.

Through her efforts and faith, she was blessed with a set of twins, followed later by a new sibling conceived naturally. Still, she continued to have a vision that she would have another baby; she already had a picture pinned on her vision board. Once again, the doctors told her it wasn't possible. Yet, two years later she was again blessed with a beautiful and healthy baby girl—looking identical to the one pinned on her board. Don't underestimate the power of a vision board!

JOURNALING

Though it may feel time consuming, or even silly, journaling is another valuable practice. Create time, as you would with any of these practices, even just five to ten minutes, four days a week (or a little more, or a little less), and write in a journal. Choose one that fits your personality and writing style, and sit in an area where you feel comfortable.

Divide the page into three sections. Use the top section to write down anything you want or feel. It can be your goals, questions, positive affirmations–anything at all. You might be surprised by what comes out, not only on the paper but also from within yourself. This section is your lead-in area, serving as a warm-up to your fitness and health goals section.

The next section will allow you to track your diet and nutrition. It should include notes on your diet, the foods you eat and at what time of day, and the foods you "cheat" with. We all have slip-ups! Write honestly about your eating habits so you can look back, when needed, and see when you were on point and when you went off track. Journaling is also a way to know which foods work and don't work for you. I stay pretty consistent on what I eat every day at every meal, but there are times when I add or remove a food, and journaling is a great way to remember how I felt, or even looked, when I altered my routine. A good journal of eating habits and foods in your diet can offer answers to questions later.

The last section should be your workout routines and the weights and reps used. By journaling these facts, you can see how you progress in strength and personal goals. It's great to look back months into a workout journal and see how you started with 25 lb (11 kg) on an exercise and progressed to 35 lb (16 kg) or increased reps with the same weight. It helps keep you motivated and excited to get to the next workout. Journaling is a peaceful release, a way to clear the mind, and a strategy for releasing pent-up emotion as you progress toward your goals.

THE POWER OF NATURE

A simple and easy way to reach your best mental state is to spend time in nature. Life gets busy, and sometimes we forget that nature can soothe us and bring us back to earth. Nature also encourages us to be active and will empower your workouts and encourage your nutritional plan. It helps quiet our minds. Nature is a wonderful setting in which to journal. Nature helps us socially. When we become too connected to our phone or the Internet, being in nature can help us reset. Begin with twenty minutes per day, maybe two or three times a week, and discover the peace and balance that being outdoors can bring. This balanced life feeling will fuel your quest to make the most progress.

Now that I've coached in you a lifestyle of fitness, nutrition, health, and well-being, you can begin to see the importance of mental fitness to your total fitness. There are many interconnecting parts to living this life that allow you to overcome your obstacles, and mental fitness is key.

DEALING WITH BURNOUT

There is a close link to obtaining the fitness, health, and nutritional results you desire and experiencing burnout along the way. You do not have to be a competitive athlete to experience this phenomenon. Burnout can occur when you are overworked, overfatigued, or overstressed–mentally or physically. I have learned to live with extreme fatigue on a daily basis, as it is a regular symptom of the disease. When you throw in the stress and wear and tear that competitive bodybuilding brings, it is almost impossible to feel totally rested. There is also a blurred line between physical and mental fatigue when dealing with MS as an athlete. So, I have to say, I am an expert in exhaustion!

The key to overcoming and dealing with mental exhaustion is to look first at the physical demands you put on your body. When the body is overfatigued, the mind is quick to follow, and vice versa. We, as athletes, seldom take a break; rather, we tend to overtrain our bodies.

I know personally how hard it is to take even one day off from the gym. I feel lost, and it breaks my routine. But that day off, and even a short daily break, can make a huge difference in my level of stress and exhaustion. This easing off the constant body drain actually helps with the mental drain.

Burnout comes from persistent stress, whether emotional or physical. Stress itself is not burnout. But when you endure extreme stress day after day, burnout is inevitable. The mind-body connection is impossible to disconnect unless you consciously put an effort into doing so.

The key is to keep a positive mind-set for as long as possible. To do that, use the tools we just discussed: create a vision board, post affirmations in your home, office, car, wherever, set time aside for meditation, or practice relaxing yoga sessions. Any time spent destressing and embracing a peaceful environment, both mentally and physically, will help you deal with mental exhaustion.

I know this all sounds like an easy answer to avoiding burnout, but finding the time and actually following through with any of this is a challenge in our fast-paced lives. I have learned, especially dealing with MS, how important taking charge of my emotions and avoiding burnout are. So I have made it a priority—something that is not a choice but a routine—to find the hour, or even the fifteen minutes, every day to settle down, unwind, and keep burnout *out* of my vocabulary. Mental fitness, like physical fitness, is a lifestyle and not a thirty-day program to success or a quick fix for results. If you want to reach your goals, you will need to adopt the same philosophy—and never quit!

 Doctor's Note

Burnout can be a real issue in MS. As long as MS patients tackle their fatigue, stress, and heat intolerance in a reasonable and safe manner, these issues may be manageable.

Stress vs. Burnout

Know the differences between stress and burnout.

Stress	Burnout
Characterized by overengagement	Characterized by disengagement
Emotions are overreactive	Emotions are blunted
Produces urgency and hyperactivity	Produces helplessness and hopelessness
Loss of energy	Leads to detachment and depression
Primary damage is physical	Primary damage is emotional

CHAPTER 3

Everyday Nutrition
Eat Right to Reach Your Goals

Let me start this chapter on nutrition with the hard honest truth: I don't like watching what I eat! The fact is, the stronger I get, the more I like to believe I am Superman, or even the Incredible Hulk–some superhuman creature who can eat food all day long without consequences. However, I am simply human, with human weaknesses. Food is my weakness. I can't get enough of it.

So, for me, nutrition is the most difficult part of my training. But I have learned that I can still love food–as long as I stick to a healthy, balanced, disease-fighting nutritional regimen, I can afford a few cheat days once in a while. Your mind is stronger than you think when it comes to disciplining yourself. When you look and feel healthy, despite your disability, it becomes easier to stick to the program and maintain it as your lifestyle. If I can do this, you can, as well.

The goal of this chapter is to provide clear nutritional guidance, address inflammation in the body, examining how to control it through nutrition and lifestyle changes, and discuss how to overcome the typical struggles of sticking with a nutritional program. For this chapter, I have worked very closely with registered dietitian Monica Pelle, R.D. She has helped me, and others with disabilities, diseases, and nutritional challenges, get on the path of healthy eating to battle our obstacles. Monica is also the director of nutrition for my MS Fitness Challenge charity, so I have tremendous respect for her knowledge and guidance.

INFLAMMATION

Inflammation is a protective response by the immune system to any type of bodily injury or infection. Inflammation is a healthy and necessary part of the immune response. It occurs when chemicals are released by your immune cells, producing swelling, redness, and pain. Initially, it is beneficial when, for example, you cut yourself and tissues need care and protection.

So what's all the fuss about? Problems occur when the immune system is triggered to release inflammatory chemicals in an ongoing and uncontrolled way. The resulting health problems can appear in any part of the body, triggering disease.

The word inflammation comes from the Latin *inflammare*, meaning "I ignite." So just imagine a fire that burns uncontrollably, creating a path of destruction. More inflammation is created in response to the existing inflammation, unless the fire is put out. Certain conditions, such as asthma, allergies, arthritis, cardiovascular disease, and autoimmune disorders, have a clear inflammatory component.

It's widely accepted, however, that chronic, low-level inflammation–sometimes called "silent" inflammation–has now been linked with diseases ranging from heart disease, diabetes, digestive disorders, cancer, and depression to

Doctor's Note

We now think that one possible reason for the worsening disability in MS over a matter of decades is that the MS brain smolders with microscopic inflammation. This inflammation is undertreated, with at least some MS treatments, and requires stronger MS treatments or additional approaches. Although not well studied, diet may be one way to control some inflammation in MS.

Alzheimer's disease. Inflammation also appears to be a key factor in accelerating the aging process, including skin aging and other outward signs of aging. Low-level inflammation can also be a roadblock for weight loss.

Inflammation and MS

One of the main issues MS sufferers must contend with is an excessive inflammatory response, which may be exacerbated by certain foods or a lifestyle that promotes inflammatory pathways. Multiple sclerosis is a disease that involves inflammation, so it seems logical to pursue treatments that reduce it. Why not try an anti-inflammatory diet and lifestyle? We'll provide a starting point.

NUTRITION AND MS

Nutrition is a major part of the battle againstMS. It has multiple facets, from the foods you eat and the liquids you drink to the supplements and herbs you add to your diet plan. Although some inflammatory diseases have diet prescriptions—a cardiac diet, for example—there is no official diet prescription for MS. However, this chapter includes common sense recommendations backed by scientific studies.

In a 2015 groundbreaking study by Riccio and Rossana published in the journal *ASN Neuro*, researchers said that the Western-style diet—characterized by red meat, sugar-sweetened drinks, fried food, low fiber, and a lack of physical exercise—produces and encourages inflammation. "Eating this type of diet over the long term creates pro-inflammatory pathways and an imbalance of our gut microbiota, which in turn affects the immune system and the ongoing inflammation in our bodies," explains Pelle.

The gut microbiota describes the microbe population living in our intestines. Our gut microbiota contains tens of trillions of microorganisms. Some are beneficial while others are harmful. Our bodies work closely with these unseen residents, trying to maintain a balance. Our nutritional intake, physical activity, medications, stress levels, and other factors, affect our gut microbial populations, which can have a huge effect on our health.

All disease begins in the gut. Hippocrates made this statement more than 2,000 years ago, and it is just as true today. It's worth noting that gut microbiota are being studied extensively and appear to be critically important in many areas of health. Multiple sclerosis may be one of those areas according to recent studies in *Scientific American* and the *Journal of Investigative Medicine*.

The previously mentioned study in *ASN Neuro* also found that nutritional intervention with anti-inflammatory foods and dietary supplements can alleviate many issues and side effects of MS, such as chronic fatigue, and side effects of drugs that affect the immune system. Despite knowing there are elements we can control, many people with disabilities do the opposite of what they should when it comes to nutrition. They may feel they are already limited, or too far from their ideal bodies, so why make the effort to eat right? Or maybe fatigue gets in the way. Just as exercise and a proper training system should be implemented with or without a disability, so should a nutrition plan.

The good news is that exercise, combined with an anti-inflammatory diet and emphasis on probiotic foods, can help decrease the body's production of inflammatory substances and promote balance in the gut microbiota. When we take control of our lifestyle, we can affect the health of our cells, and the population of our gut microbiota, thereby altering our immune system and chronic inflammatory disease.

The OptimalBody approach to nutrition is a balanced method of fueling your body for maximum physical and mental strength. Poor nutrition depletes your body of strength and energy. Optimal nutrition propels your body forward to meet life's challenges and overcome its obstacles. The Optimal-Body approach combines movement and muscle toning with a diet of anti-inflammatory foods and supplements, ensuring positive results.

 Doctor's Note

Diet is clearly important for people dealing with multiple sclerosis. We know that salt, and certain fats and spices, influence inflammation (as seen in animal studies). We know that vitamin D supplementation, or diets rich in vitamin D, is helpful in controlling MS activity. Many of my patients who start diets designed for MS feel better and seem to be more stable neurologically. Unfortunately, this is hard to study scientifically so we may never know how good any given diet is for MS.

 Doctor's Note

For MS, diet not only affects disease activity but also its symptoms. Fatigue increases with high-sugar, high-fat diets, as well as with alcohol. Foods rich in magnesium can help with spasticity and pain. Obesity is a significant problem for people with disability, and a good diet can help reduce weight to improve mobility and other weight-associated symptoms.

ADDRESSING INFLAMMATION WITH DIET AND LIFESTYLE

We've established a link between disease and inflammation, and research suggesting a total diet and lifestyle approach is one of the best prescriptions for reducing inflammation and other risk factors for disease. This basic starting point allows our bodies to heal, repair, and rebuild.

One of the biggest factors that helps control inflammation is the food you eat. Certain foods promote inflammation, while others stop it. There is no one-size-fits-all anti-inflammatory diet. In a nutshell, to move toward an anti-inflammatory diet, we primarily move away from the overly processed Standard American Diet (appropriately called SAD), and move toward the ancient eating patterns of the Mediterranean diet.

A Mediterranean diet includes:

✓ Beans

✓ Fish

✓ Fresh fruits and vegetables

✓ Herbs

✓ Nuts and seeds

✓ Olive oil

✓ Whole grains

– Limited amounts of red meat and dairy

✗ No artificial chemicals

Doctor's Note

MS doctors believe that omega-3 fatty acids, found in many of the foods typical of the Mediterranean diet, help fight inflammation in MS.

Numerous resources promote anti-inflammatory eating, and each has its own spin. One noted expert is Andrew Weil, M.D., whose anti-inflammatory food pyramid is an excellent dietary guide. Our dietitian, Monica Pelle, R.D., adheres to similar recommendations in her lists of anti-inflammatory foods that follow. Her diet recommendations focus on plant-based foods, because phytochemicals–natural chemicals found in the plants–are believed to help reduce inflammation. Such anti-inflammatory foods can regulate the immune system and change the way inflammation affects our bodies and our lives.

Recommended Anti-Inflammatory Foods

The following information provides an excellent starting point for identifying anti-inflammatory foods and beverages to incorporate into your nutrition plan. Use this practical guide to create meal plans according to your tastes, tolerances, and preferences. There is a trial-and-error phase when trying new, healing foods. As you get the processed junk out, your palate will adapt. Most people come to crave real food as they eliminate inflammation-causing foods.

As with other lifestyle changes, an anti-inflammatory diet is not meant to be a short-term eating plan. Rather, it is an ideal nutritional foundation for every family member, every day. Thinking about it less as a special diet and more as a nutritious, family-friendly way of eating may help you integrate it into your routine more easily. The more anti-inflammatory choices you make, the more you help your body maintain optimum health.

In addition to influencing inflammation, this style of eating provides steady energy, vitamins, minerals, omega-3 fatty acids, dietary fiber, and protective phytonutrients. Good nutrition is crucial to the health and function of every cell in your body. We can see the connection and significance of both diet and exercise in the prevention or progression of disease.

Foods to Avoid

We've just looked at recommended foods that can help strengthen and heal your body. For best results on the OptimalBody program, also avoid foods that create barriers on your road to fitness. Those barriers may include inflammation, pain, fatigue, disease, dysfunction, mood swings, depression, anxiety, weight gain, and feelings of failure.

Remember, perfection is not necessary. Balance, not deprivation, is the goal. Consistently avoiding the foods on page 42 in favor of more energizing and healing foods will help you reach your goals.

Doctor's Note

There is no one best diet for MS. Try to find a healthy diet you enjoy that adds value to your quality of life. Many MS patients who modify their diet eliminate gluten or choose a Paleo diet. As long as you tolerate these changes and, hopefully, feel better as well, these are all fine diets.

Doctor's Note

Remember to balance all these issues and concepts when designing a diet for yourself. The most important thing to keep in mind is how good you feel over time on any particular diet.

Healing Anti-Inflammatory Foods

Food group and serving recommendations	Guidance	Suggested foods
VEGETABLES **Servings:** On an anti-inflammatory meal plan, the majority of daily food servings comes from vegetables; a minimum of 4 to 5 servings per day. 1 serving = 2 cups (142 g) leafy greens; ½ cup (~60 g, depending on the vegetable) of vegetables cooked, raw, or juiced	• Choose a wide range of colors. • Try to include raw servings daily. • Steam or boil green vegetables in a little water, but do not overcook to avoid losing vitamin content. • Eat cruciferous (cabbage family) vegetables regularly. • Eat plenty of green leafy vegetables. • Choose organic when possible. Make note of the Dirty Dozen (most pesticide-contaminated foods) at www.ewg.org to determine which are best to buy organic.	Artichokes Asparagus Beets Bell peppers Broccoli Brussels sprouts Cabbage Carrots Cauliflower Celery Cucumbers Garlic Green beans Green leafy vegetables: dark green, leafy lettuce, swiss chard, spinach, kale, collard greens, bok choy, micro greens Jicama Mushrooms Onions Pumpkin Sea vegetables Shiitake mushrooms Squash Sugar snap peas Sweet potatoes Tomato Zucchini

Food group and serving recommendations	Guidance	Suggested foods
FRUITS **Servings:** 3 servings per day. 1 serving = 1 medium piece; ½ cup (~75 g depending on the fruit) diced fruit; ¼ cup (grams vary) organic dried fruit with no added sugar	• Choose a wide range of colors. • Choose fruits that are fresh and in season, or frozen. • Choose organic when possible. Make note of the Dirty Dozen (most pesticide-contaminated foods) at www.ewg.org to determine which are best to buy organic. • All fruits in this list are lower in glycemic load (how they raise blood sugar levels) than other fruits.	Apples Berries: blackberries, blueberries, boysenberries, cranberries, raspberries, strawberries Cherries Lemon Lime Oranges Pears Pineapple Pink grapefruit Pomegranate Red grapes
WHOLE GRAINS **Servings:** 3 to 5 servings per day. 1 serving = ½ cup (~100 g depending on the grain) cooked grains **Pasta:** 2 to 3 servings per week; 1 pasta serving = ½ cup (~70 g)	• A gluten-free diet may be beneficial. Not all whole grains listed are gluten-free. • Focus on grains (with a low glycemic load) that are less refined, less processed, high in fiber, slowly digested. • Reduce your consumption of foods made with wheat flour and sugar, especially bread and most packaged snack foods. • Eat more whole grains in which the grain is intact, such as brown rice. These are preferable to whole-wheat flour products, which have roughly the same glycemic index (blood sugar impact) as white flour products. • Cook pasta al dente and eat it in moderation.	Amaranth Barley Basmati rice Brown rice Buckwheat Millet Quinoa Spelt Steel-cut oats Wild rice

Food group and serving recommendations	Guidance	Suggested foods
PROTEIN-RICH FOODS **Meat, Poultry, Fish, and Eggs** **Servings:** 2 to 6 servings per week; 1 serving = 4 oz (115 g) fish, turkey, or chicken	• Eat lean protein sources, such as chicken, and avoid red meat. • Decrease consumption of animal protein and balance it with vegetable protein. • Choose grass-fed lean meats that are free of preservatives, antibiotics, growth hormones, nitrates, or coloring. • Choose organic when possible.	Albacore tuna (low-mercury brands available) Alaskan halibut Anchovies Herring Mackerel Omega-3-enriched eggs Sardines (packed in water or olive oil) Skinless chicken breast Skinless turkey breast Trout Wild salmon (canned, fresh, or frozen)
Beans and Legumes A note: Beans, legumes, and organic soy are not tolerated by everyone. Listen to your body. **General recommendations for servings:** Beans and legumes: 1 to 2 servings per day; 1 serving = ½ cup (~115 g) Organic soy: 1 to 2 servings per day, as tolerated; 1 serving = ½ cup (80 g) cooked edamame; ½ cup (126 g) tofu or tempeh; 1 oz (28 g) soy nuts	• These foods are a great way to eat more vegetable protein on a daily basis. • Eat them whole or puréed into spreads, such as hummus. • Choose organic whole soy foods. Avoid heavily processed soy.	Beans: adzuki, black, cannellini, fava, garbanzo (chickpeas), kidney, lima, mung, navy, pinto Black-eyed peas Edamame (boiled soybeans) Soy (organic) Soy nuts Tempeh Tofu

Food group and serving recommendations	Guidance	Suggested foods
HEALTHY FATS **Servings:** 5 to 7 servings per day; 1 serving = 1 teaspoon (5 ml) oil; 2 tablespoons (~about 16 g depending on the type of nut), nut butters, or seeds; 2 tablespoons (28 g) avocado	• Ideally, choose nuts and seeds that are raw and unsalted. • Watch portion sizes to prevent weight gain. Consume daily.	Avocados Cold-pressed sesame oil Extra-virgin olive oil Nuts and nut butters (no sugar added): almonds, cashews, pecans, walnuts Organic expeller-pressed canola oil, coconut oil, grapeseed oil Seeds and butters (no sugar added): chia, flaxseed, hemp, pumpkin/pepita, sesame, sunflower
DAIRY AND NON-DAIRY ALTERNATIVES **Servings:** High-quality natural cheeses in moderation; 1 serving = 1 to 2 oz (28 to 55 g) per week; limit organic cow's milk to 1 to 2 cups (235 to 475 ml) per week. Some people do not tolerate cow's milk products at all.	• Cut back on cow's milk dairy and try plant-based alternatives, such as unsweetened nut milks (almond, coconut, cashew). There are many recipes for homemade options; when purchasing from a store, avoid carrageenan on the ingredients list. • Small amounts of full-fat dairy are preferable to non-fat and low-fat alternatives. • Choose probiotic yogurts and non-dairy milks with no added sugar.	Goat's milk or sheep's milk feta Goat's milk yogurt Jarlsberg Manchego Organic plain probiotic yogurt Organic soy milk Parmesan Romano Swiss Unsweetened almond milk Unsweetened coconut milk Unsweetened kefir

Food group and serving recommendations	Guidance	Suggested foods
HERBS AND SPICES **Servings:** Add to foods and beverages throughout the day in unlimited amounts.	• Use a variety of herbs and spices to season food. • Replace salt, sugar, and added fat by boosting flavor.	Basil Chile peppers Chives Cilantro Cinnamon Citrus zest Curry powder Dill Ginger Mint Oregano Parsley Rosemary Thyme Turmeric
BEVERAGES **Servings:** Tea: 2 to 4 cups (475 to 946 ml each) per day Alcohol: to 1 to 2 glasses (5 to 10 oz or 150 to 285 ml each) per day Daily fluid intake: To estimate general daily fluid goals, divide your body weight in pounds (kg) by 2. For example, a 150-lb (68 kg) person = 75 oz (2.2 L) of fluids.	• Drink tea instead of coffee. • If you drink alcohol, limit it; if you don't drink alcohol now, avoid picking up the habit. • Drink filtered water throughout the day. • Choose glass or stainless steel water bottles over plastic. Plastic's chemicals migrate into foods and beverages.	Bone broth Chicory root coffee Fresh squeezed lemon or lime in water Good-quality white, green, or oolong tea Kombucha with less than ½ teaspoon of sugar per serving Organic red wine (if you choose to drink alcohol) Other beneficial teas: cinnamon, ginger, licorice, peppermint, roasted dandelion root Plain filtered water Sparkling water, such as Pellegrino

Food group and serving recommendations	Guidance	Suggested foods
SWEET TREATS **Servings:** Enjoy plain dark chocolate in moderation, 1 oz (28 g) a few times per week; stevia in unlimited quantities; and xylitol, as tolerated. Some people are sensitive to loose stools with xylitol and others eat it daily without problem. Listen to your body. Use natural sweeteners sparingly. They are not required as part of a healthy diet and contribute to inflammation, but are preferable to refined sugars.	• Experiment with natural sweeteners, such as coconut palm sugar, lucuma powder, raw honey, and Medjool dates. Even these are inflammatory, but preferable to regular sugar. • For zero-calorie sweetness, avoid artificial sweeteners and choose sweeteners, such as stevia and xylitol. Stevia is the gold standard for natural non-caloric sweeteners. Some people are sensitive to xylitol and may experience loose stools. • Choose naturally sweet desserts.	Non-GMO xylitol Plain, dark chocolate (minimum 70% cocoa content) Stevia

Food group and serving recommendations	Guidance	Suggested foods
PROBIOTIC FOODS **Servings:** Consuming probiotic-rich foods daily is a good practice. Consider: 1 cup (230 g) yogurt ½ cup (83 g) tempeh ½ cup (120 ml) kefir ¼ cup (36 g) sauerkraut or fermented vegetables 1 cup (8 oz or 235 ml) chicory root coffee 1 cup (8 oz or 235 ml) kombucha	• Probiotic foods repopulate your gut microbiota with beneficial bacteria, crowd out candida (yeast), restore stomach acidity, and boost your immune system. • Avoid yogurts that claim to be probiotic but don't list the specific strains of bacteria on the packaging. • Buy the "raw" or "unpasteurized" forms of sauerkraut and kimchi, otherwise, the beneficial bacteria are destroyed in processing. Health food stores often sell these items. • Some probiotics contain prebiotics, non-digestible foods that feed the probiotics. Inulin is one example. Chicory coffee is also a good source of inulin, as well as being caffeine free.	Homemade fermented vegetables Kimchi Organic tempeh Plain organic yogurt Sauerkraut Unsweetened kefir
SUPPLEMENTS	• The majority of nutritional needs are best met consuming fresh, wholesome foods. • Nutritional gaps can be filled with high-quality supplements. • Supplements are not an alternative to a healthy diet. You should still maintain a variety and balance.	**Common daily needs are:** Anti-inflammatory substances, such as turmeric and ginger Coenzyme Q_{10} Fish oil for omega-3s (both EPA and DHA) Key antioxidants Multivitamin/multi-mineral Probiotics Vitamin D_3

Foods to Limit or Avoid

Guidance	Avoid these foods
Minimize processed foods and refined grains.	Bread, chips, corn chips, and products made with white flour, such as bagels, crackers, and pretzels, french fries, pizza, white pasta, white rice
Minimize saturated fats and trans fats because they damage the cells that line blood vessels.	Cream, ice cream, high-fat cheeses, and fried foods; margarine, vegetable shortening, and all products listing them as ingredients
Limit processed and high-fat meats.	Non-grass-fed beef, fast food, hot dogs, lamb, lunch meats, pork, sausages
Avoid sugary foods and beverages.	Candy, corn syrup, pastries, presweetened cereals, sodas, sweetened beverages
Avoid inflammatory foods.	As a general rule, if it contains refined flour or sugar, or is a high-fat meat, it will be pro-inflammatory.

 Doctor's Note

- A sugar crash can also strongly influence fatigue, which is an especially common symptom in MS.

- Sugary drinks, such as sodas, are important to avoid because they are calorie rich, highly inflammatory, and drastically promote weight gain in the long term.

An Important Note on Sugar

Sugar can be one of the most significant barriers for eating right to reach your goals. Consuming sugar, especially processed sugar, lights an immediate inflammatory fire in your body. A growing body of scientific evidence reveals sugar's contribution to obesity, diabetes, heart disease, stroke, high blood pressure, high cholesterol and triglycerides, cancer, candida, inflammation throughout the body, mood swings, and as a threat to the immune system. It also affects your gut microbiota by feeding yeast and crowding out good bacteria. A 2014 study published in the *Journal of the American Medical Association* [*JAMA*] showed that too much added sugar in your diet can significantly increase your risk of dying from cardiovascular disease.

Another study found that eating high-glycemic foods (foods that raise blood sugar quickly) can create a sharp crash in blood sugar levels that leads to overeating at the next meal. And here's the mind-blower: Researchers noticed that the rapid drop in blood sugar lit up the region of the brain connected to addictive behaviors. This gives credibility to the idea that we can develop an actual addiction to sugar-laden foods. Because of sugar's huge impact on heart health, the American Heart Association (AHA) has set guidelines for its intake. AHA recommends the following for added sugars:

- **No more than 6 teaspoons (24 g) or 100 calories a day for women**
- **No more than 9 teaspoons (36 g) or 150 calories a day for men**

What counts as added sugar? Added sugars are sugars and syrups added to foods or beverages when they're processed or prepared. Added sugars contribute additional calories and zero nutrients to food. Naturally occurring sugars are found in certain foods, such as fruit (fructose) and milk (lactose).

Most American adults consume about 22 teaspoons (88 g) of added sugar a day. That's two to four times the AHA-recommended daily intake! Sugar-sweetened beverages are the largest source of added sugars in the American diet. A can of regular soda packs about 9 teaspoons (about 35 g) of added sugars—an entire day's worth of added sugar. Other major sources are candy, cookies, ice cream, sweetened yogurt, and cereals. Therefore, keeping tabs on your sugar consumption is an important part of a healthy lifestyle.

Many people consume much more sugar than they realize. Next time you eat a packaged food, check the nutrition facts panel. The line for sugars contains both the natural and added types as total grams of sugar. The format for this label hasn't changed in twenty years, but it may be changing soon, making added sugars easier to detect.

To tell whether a processed food contains added sugars, look at the list of ingredients. Sugar has many other names:

- **Ingredients ending in "-ose," such as maltose, dextrose, or sucrose**
- **Barley malt**
- **Cane juice**
- **Cane sugar, beet sugar, or raw sugar**
- **Corn sweetener, corn syrup, or high-fructose corn syrup**
- **Fruit juice concentrate**
- **Molasses**
- **Sugar cane syrup**

For sugar alternatives, we tend to seek out synthetic artificial sweeteners, such as aspartame and Splenda. These synthetically produced alternatives will only harm your health. The good news is there are plenty of natural sugar alternatives. With the exception of stevia, these lower-glycemic sweeteners still count as sugar intake, so moderation is needed. Following are some of the most beneficial natural sugars you can find.

Stevia: An herb native to South America, stevia is 300 times sweeter than sugar. It has zero calories and no glycemic impact. This is my number one pick for a healthy sweetener. You can purchase both organic liquid and powder stevia from most stores now. You can use it to sweeten your coffee, tea, and smoothies. If baking with stevia, it's best to use a recipe that's actually written to use stevia rather than regular sugar. Allow your palate time to adjust to it. It's worth it!

Coconut palm sugar: Produced from the sap of the coconut palm tree, coconut sugar is nutritious and has a lower score on the glycemic index. It tastes similar to brown sugar but is slightly richer. You can substitute coconut sugar for traditional sugar.

Raw honey: Always opt for raw honey to ensure you are getting all of its valuable nutrients and enzymes. Raw and local honey is also good for seasonal allergies. There is nothing beneficial about processed honey.

Lucuma powder: Touted as a superfood, it has a uniquely sweet and maple-like taste. It's perfect for sweetening beverages, smoothies, yogurt, granola, pudding, or homemade ice cream, as well as for baking cakes, cookies, and pies.

Medjool dates: These can be used to sweeten smoothies, and for cooking and baking for a touch of sweetness. Additionally they pack fiber, potassium, magnesium, B vitamins, calcium, and phosphorous.

To manage your sugar intake, follow these suggestions:

- Experiment with natural sweeteners to find one you like.
- Reduce or eliminate soda, sports and energy drinks, as well as enhanced waters, sweetened teas, and sugary coffee drinks.
- Cut back on the amount of sugar added to things you eat or drink regularly, such as cereal, coffee, or tea.
- Avoid adding sugar to cereal or oatmeal; try fresh fruit (oranges, cherries, or strawberries) instead.
- Avoid adding sugar in recipes; use extracts, such as almond, vanilla, orange, or lemon.
- Enhance foods with spices instead of sugar. Try allspice, cinnamon, ginger, or nutmeg.
- Buy fresh fruits or fruits canned in water or natural juice; avoid fruit canned in syrup.

With all these natural sugar alternatives readily available, it's getting easier to reduce total sugar intake while still enjoying tasty, healthier options. The keys to success are to monitor how much sugar you consume and switching to healthier options when you do enjoy a sweet treat–in moderation.

LIVING AN ANTI-INFLAMMATORY LIFESTYLE

Small, gradual changes are typically easier for the body to adapt to, more sustainable, and can make you less likely to revert to your old ways. So, rather than trying to adopt all these suggestions overnight, think about how you can adopt this lifestyle one step at a time.

What we eat and drink either feeds disease or fights it.

Healthy lifestyle habits that help reduce inflammation include:

- **Exercising regularly.** Physical exercise influences the quality of life and may stimulate the production of anti-inflammatory cytokines. A 2015 study by P.D. Lopinizi published in the journal *Physiology & Behavior* showed that establishing a daily routine of moderate to vigorous physical activity is better at reducing inflammation than intermittent movement throughout the week.
- **Not smoking.** The effects of cigarette smoking on the immune system are far reaching and complex. Smoking not only creates inflammation but also suppresses the immune system.
- **Reducing toxin load.** This means reducing chemicals we're exposed to both by what we put on, and in, our bodies. To help, use only natural cleaning products, eat whole foods without added preservatives, try therapeutic essential oils, and reduce the plastics you eat and drink from.

- **Maintaining a healthy weight.** Fat cells produce inflammatory chemicals at a rate far greater than other cells. Having a high body mass index before age 20 is associated with increased risk for multiple sclerosis in both men and women.

- **Minimizing stress.** This even includes managing hurt feelings. A 2001 study (Slavich et al.) published in the *Proceedings of the National Academy of Sciences of the United States of America*, showed social stresses, such as feeling rejected, increased inflammatory markers in people.

- **Getting quality sleep.** People who sleep poorly or do not get enough sleep have higher levels of inflammation.

- **Consuming an anti-inflammatory diet.** What we eat and drink either feeds disease or fights it.

In summary, our goal is to make the OptimalBody approach to nutrition a style of eating and living that is realistic and sustainable. It's common to have days when you eat a combination of inflammatory and anti-inflammatory foods. It's nearly impossible to avoid all inflammatory foods all the time. The primary goal is to bring your diet into balance. Take the first steps: Decrease the foods that contribute to disease and increase the healing foods so the overall effect of your diet is anti-inflammatory. To accomplish this, meal planning and food forethought are needed. It takes energy to plan, shop, and prepare the foods your body needs. Keeping a well-stocked fridge and pantry help make it easier. When you avoid those foods known to make you feel tired, sick, and mentally low, you'll feel empowered to take control.

MEAL PLANNING

Now that you know which foods to enjoy and which foods to avoid, you can begin to build your meal plan. Being told what to eat at every meal won't empower you to gain the skills to manage a healthy diet properly. The people who are most successful with healthy eating over the long term go through the process of finding pleasure in the foods that lead them to health. The journey is exciting and rewarding.

Fuel your journey, and you will reach your destination.

Take it one step at a time, one meal at a time. Use your journal or mobile app to document what works for you and what doesn't. The app can also help you see whether you're hitting your personal nutritional targets. Look online: There are meal-planning websites to help organize your weekly plans and countless recipes available. Fitness tracker logging apps or online tools, such as MyFitnessPal (MyFitnessPal.com), can help with portion sizes appropriate for your body and are backed by health professionals and nutritionists. Eat regular meals (especially breakfast) and snacks throughout the day to maintain blood sugar levels and stimulate metabolism. And remember, proper nutrition is a must on your road to fitness. You can't outwork a poor diet. Fuel your journey, and you will reach your destination.

Sample Meal Plan for an Anti-inflammatory Diet

Day 1	Day 2	Day 3
Breakfast Super greens smoothie: blend frozen berries, organic kale, water, and vegetarian protein powder	**Breakfast** Spinach and mushroom frittata	**Breakfast** Oatmeal: old-fashioned oats, cinnamon, walnuts, and almond milk
Lunch Asian bowl: brown rice, vegetables, and chicken	**Lunch** Tuna salad on whole-grain bread with apple slices	**Lunch** Lentil soup, mixed greens salad, and flax crackers
Dinner Turkey chili and muffin made with almond flour	**Dinner** Wild salmon, quinoa, sautéed zucchini, and garlic	**Dinner** Stuffed bell peppers (stuffed with quinoa and grass-fed ground beef)
Snack Organic Greek yogurt with sunflower seeds	**Snack** Carrots and hummus; dark chocolate (70 percent cocoa)	**Snack** Organic celery and apple slices with almond butter
Beverage In addition to filtered water, roasted dandelion root tea	**Beverage** In addition to filtered water, ginger lemonade (made with freshly grated ginger and lemon juice and sweetened with stevia)	**Beverage** In addition to filtered water, green tea

Eating Before and After Exercise

Nutrition plays an important role in your exercise performance. Without adequate carbohydrates and fluid, you'll quickly become fatigued. Protein rebuilds muscles. Without these three fundamental elements, plus adequate vitamins and minerals, you will struggle to tap into your potential. If you have a poor diet, expect poor performance. Poor nutrition can also lead to injury and poor recovery, both of which can hinder your ability to continue your fitness plan.

Our bodies are like machines in some ways: Put quality fuel into the engine, and it will be primed for excellent performance. However, if you put lesser-quality fuel into the engine, performance can suffer. That's why you need to pay close attention to when and what you're eating before, during, and after a workout.

> Nutrition plays an important role in your exercise performance.

As with all nutrition plans, there are several variables to consider. Portions and percentages of foods needed vary based on gender, body weight, and intensity, type, and length of your workout. Whether you choose a meal or snack before and after a workout largely depends on your plan for the day. With a little preparation and planning, optimum results can be achieved. With the following guidelines, you can customize a plan that works best for you. As always, reach for additional support as needed. A registered dietitian can help you develop a structured plan based on your unique needs. With so many aspects out of our control, nutrition is a performance variable you can control. Take advantage of it!

Make the Most of Your Workout

Pre-Workout Meal Guidelines

- Choose easily digested carbohydrates and low-fat foods for quicker digestion.
- Avoid starting a workout when you're starved or stuffed.
- Pay attention to whole foods, they are an important energy source. Avoid processed foods.
- Eat thirty to sixty minutes before beginning a cardio workout, and eat 75 to 100 percent carbohydrates.
- Eat one to two hours before beginning a strength-training workout, and eat 75 percent carbs and 25 percent protein.
- Eat carbs thirty to sixty minutes prior to workouts that contain both strength-training and cardio. Eat protein within two hours prior.
- Drink plenty of water for proper hydration.

Pre-Workout Fuel Ideas

- Banana and coconut milk
- Carrots and hummus
- Dried fruit with no added sugar or preservatives
- Greek yogurt and fruit
- Hardboiled egg and slice of whole-grain toast
- Oatmeal with apples
- Organic unsweetened applesauce with cinnamon
- Roasted sweet potatoes
- Super green smoothie with fruit, greens, and protein powder
- Whole-grain cereal and almond milk
- Whole-grain waffle with berries

Ideas during Workout

- Water
- Organic fruit juice diluted in water

Guidelines during Workout

- Drink plenty of water, at least 4 oz (120 ml) for every twenty minutes of exercise. Perspiration and exertion deplete the body of fluids necessary for optimal performance and lead to dehydration.
- There is no need to replace carbohydrates during a workout unless the exercise lasts more than ninety minutes and is hard and continuous. When this happens, drink 100 percent fruit juice diluted in water to provide fuel and water to the muscles being exercised.

Post-Workout Meal Guidelines

The longer we wait to eat something, the longer it takes to recover. The enzymes that help the body resynthesize muscle glycogen and build muscle are most active in that first fifteen minutes after a workout. Realistically, the goal is to eat within a one-hour post-workout window.

- Eat quality protein (10 to 20 grams) within fifteen to thirty minutes after working out. Whole foods are best, but healthy bars and shakes are an easy option.
- Strength workout: Protein and carbs repair muscles and replenish glycogen stores.
- Cardio workout: Replace glycogen (stored carbohydrates) lost during workout with complex carbohydrates, such as sweet potatoes, brown rice, quinoa, or oatmeal.
- Rehydrate with fluids. The average workout does not demand the extra calories and electrolytes in sports drinks, not to mention artificial coloring and junky sweeteners. Coconut water is a great alternative to sports drinks for electrolyte balance.

Post-Workout Recovery Meal Ideas

- Bean burrito: organic corn tortilla filled with black beans, Greek yogurt, and salsa
- Hummus and whole-grain crackers
- Organic edamame
- Protein bar: 10 to 20 grams of protein, fewer than 5 grams of sugar
- Protein pancakes: lots of recipes out there for all diets
- Protein shake: blend one scoop protein powder, one banana, and 8 ounces (235 ml) water
- Sandwich: chicken; turkey; peanut butter and jelly; egg; salmon or tuna on whole-grain bread with veggies
- Spinach and feta egg scramble
- Stir-fried chicken and vegetables over brown rice or quinoa
- Super green smoothie with protein powder
- Veggie omelet and slice of whole-grain toast

One of the best tips I can give you is never start a workout on an empty stomach, especially in the morning. It's a common practice for people to wake up early, skip breakfast, and jump right on the treadmill. You're not doing yourself any favors by going in empty. Training on an empty stomach, or in a state of fasting, can cause you to lose muscle you have worked so hard to create. The benefits of eating before exercise, particularly carbs and protein, far outweigh any perceived benefits from fasting. Having these substances available as fuel will limit protein loss and thus maintain muscle mass, increase performance, and help the body use more fat after the workout.

HEALTHY EATING ON A BUDGET

Motivation, energy, and strength are not the only potential barriers on your road to fitness. Financial barriers are a common reality, especially if you've had several medical issues. A healthy diet can be more expensive. Fish and fresh fruits and vegetables can be particularly pricey. However, eating healthy on a budget is possible with the right approach. It would be unwise to skimp on the very investment that guarantees a great return. My grandmother used to say, "You can pay at the grocery store, or you can pay at the doctor's office." She was proof of the preventive effects a healthy diet can have and the value of investing in fresh, wholesome food–not to mention your own nutrition and wellness. Follow these tips for eating healthy on a budget:

• Cook several portions of a dish and freeze some. This also saves you the effort of preparing meals every day.

• Use frozen fruits and vegetables; they are often cheaper than fresh produce and are smart nutritional choices.

• Buy fresh fruit and vegetables in season, when they are usually cheaper.

• Plan some vegetarian meals. Beans and lentils are cheaper than meat.

• Choose canned wild salmon as it is an affordable protein and source of omega-3 fatty acids.

• Cut down on sugary drinks, junk food, and alcohol to make room in your budget for more quality food purchases.

• Map out your weekly meals ahead of time. Food in the trash equals money in the trash. Before you buy more food, take stock of what you have on hand and plan meals around that. Planning ahead will also help you eat out less–a big money and health saver.

Meal planning, dieting, healthy eating, and smart nutrition all boil down to one thing: a philosophy combined with a program. Willpower alone does not guarantee success. Living a lifestyle that includes a nutritionally sound regimen brings you that much closer to your goals. Having a disability that complicates your life or is burdensome adds another dimension to your plan, but it does not make it impossible. I'm living proof! The OptimalBody nutritional methodology works because it puts all the mechanisms in place for you to succeed. Once you make the decision to change the course of your disability to one that you control, following the sound guidance to a healthier OptimalBody lifestyle will be as normal as showering each day. You can do this!

MUST-HAVE MIND-SETS FOR LONG-TERM SUCCESS

Now that you know which foods can support your success, let's look at the food-related mind-sets that need to accompany these foods. Whether we're trying to eat healthier, get fit, lose weight, or change any other behavior, we need to attach a mind-set to it. The mind-set with which you approach your diet will determine whether your journey is filled with success or roadblocks. Developing a long-term healthy lifestyle is hard enough, so remove unnecessary roadblocks from the start.

Set Your Mind for Success

• Kick negative thoughts to the curb, and instead, think about the possibilities ahead.

• Ditch perfection.

• Learn to fish.

• Reach out for support.

• Find pleasure in the foods that lead you to health.

Let's start by kicking a few self-defeating thoughts to the curb. Negative mind-sets will not help you achieve a healthier lifestyle. Replace negative thinking with thoughts that will help you stay the course. Think about possibility, capability, and your potential for achieving what you set your mind to. These thoughts will help you tap into your motivation and inspiration. When you combine positive mind-sets and a sense of what's realistic in your life, you get tremendous potential for a strategy that you can actually be successful with for the long run.

> Think about possibility, capability, and your potential for achieving what you set your mind to.

Let's look at some additional must-have mind-sets that are crucial as you embark on the OptimalBody approach to nutrition.

Must-Have Mind-Sets about Nutrition

Avoid Negative Mind-Sets	Replace Negative Thoughts with Positive, Empowering Thoughts
• "I don't have the time, money, or energy to prepare healthy food on a regular basis." • "I don't like food that's good for me." • "I've tried diets before, and I couldn't stick with them."	• "I can and will learn how to change my diet." • "My health is important enough to keep trying." • "I can find a way, or I can find an excuse. I choose to find a way."

Ditch Perfection

Perfectionism is one of the greatest barriers to long-term behavior change. Perfectionist mind-sets tend to be all or nothing—on a diet or off a diet, deprivation or excess, perfection or failure. These extremes do not help you because life is a series of progressions and regressions. Smooth times and chaotic times. You'll go on vacation, celebrate holidays, eat treats, get sick, juggle family emergencies, and more. Expect the unexpected while you work to improve your health.

Maintaining a healthy diet is a life-long process, and being prepared for the ups and downs is crucial to success. Just remember, this process is designed to train your brain and your body for balance. Patiently keep pressing the reset button. You're not trying to be perfect. Rather, you're trying to make progress. Keep repeating this mantra, "Progress, not perfection." Give yourself a pat on the back for making even the smallest step toward balance, and then make another step each day.

Learn to Fish

"Give a man a fish and you feed him for a day. Teach a man to fish and you feed him for a lifetime" is a well-known Chinese proverb. Many people think they want the fish—in other words, someone to tell them exactly what and how much to eat daily. But there are several flaws in that approach. It's not a sustainable practice to follow daily eating instructions, and you won't "learn to fish" in the process. Any nutrition approach that is centered on your best interests is designed to empower you, to create a sense of capability and ownership. With self-knowledge and personal responsibility, you'll be able to assess where you are on the path and where you need to go when challenges arise.

Statements from someone learning to fish, someone taking control of their own nutrition plan, sound like this:

- "I found a great mobile app for meal planning."
- "I researched some recipes that support my nutrition goals."
- "I tossed out all the junk food that is not supporting my health."
- "I figured out a realistic way to divide the grocery shopping, cooking, and cleanup in my family."

Statements such as these are telltale signs that people are taking ownership of the way they feed themselves and becoming problem solvers. Taking ownership can be overwhelming when you don't know where to start, or you're not feeling well physically or mentally. The good news is that improving your nutrition does not have to be a solo journey.

Reach Out for Support

As you begin your road to fitness or even along the way, never be afraid to ask for support. There are endless support streams to tap into.

Health professionals: Don't be afraid to get short- or long-term support from health professionals. Investing in your wellness with an expert can be life changing. In my own wellness journey, I've worked with holistic health practitioners, including acupuncturists, chiropractors, massage therapists, dietitians, and naturopaths. Investing in the right help can actually save you money in the long term. Look for practitioners who want to teach you to empower yourself.

Doctor's Note

MS doctors know a lot about medicines and how to manage MS medically, but not as much about diets. Seek the counsel of dietitians, other MS patients, MS groups, and people close to you to determine what diet you think is best for you. Break diets down to what you specifically want: a diet to help with reducing relapse risk or symptoms, such as fatigue, pain, sensory problems, or immobility.

Friends, family, community, and employers: Enlist people you can lean on when you need encouragement for healthy eating. They don't need to share your goals. Instead, they can simply cheer you on, ask you for progress updates, or encourage you to talk about how you're feeling today. You can also engage in online communities for extra support, accountability, and guidance from others going through a similar process. Social media is a great way to find support, motivation, and inspiration from like-minded people. And it's free! Instagram, Pinterest, and Facebook all have great resources for recipes, people passionate about health, and attractive food photos that can inspire you to try something new. Your employer, and even health insurance provider, may offer free coaching from health professionals. Employee Assistance Programs are highly underutilized in the workplace, but they are very common support tools offered by employers. When you start to investigate the lines of support in your benefits package, you may be surprised at the support tools you have at your fingertips.

Support yourself: We can all be our own worst enemy. A lot of that is related to our mind-set. The goal is to avoid self-sabotage to the extent possible. Avoid the failure syndrome trap. This syndrome is typically caused by a harsh judgment of your "mistakes" and the subsequent stream of negative feelings you experience: anger, despair, hopelessness, and numbness. These negative feelings can lead to avoidance. I'll do something about it–tomorrow. This prevents action for problem solving today. Confront challenges as they arise, even if you take only a small step.

Find Pleasure in Healthy Foods

Most people can do anything for the short term. They can white-knuckle it through restrictive diets, desperately awaiting the day they're over. Our biggest challenge is to find pleasure consistently in the choices that lead us to nutritional balance. Only when we find pleasure in balancing our nutritional needs does it become likely we will maintain these healthy habits for a lifetime. Some of the most delicious foods on the planet are good for you. Sometimes it's a matter of training your palate; other times it's a matter of training your mind.

A key reason for failure is that we embark on dietary changes that deprive us of all our likes. We see the process as all or nothing–and deprivation always leads to excess. A better strategy is to make adjustments over time, as opposed to eliminating everything overnight. Make room for treats and old favorites, as well as healthier alternatives you may like even better. For example, my family switched from refined wheat pasta to brown rice pasta and never missed it. I've experimented with almond flour and made some of the best muffins and cookies I've ever had. The possibilities are endless.

A friend once shared her observation that any time she feels like she can't stop eating a food, she knows it's a fake food.

Those processed foods loaded with fat, salt, refined sugars and carbs, artificial sweeteners, and other chemicals that are actually designed for addiction, engineered to trick your brain into wanting more. Though we do receive short-term pleasure from eating lots of these foods, they are the same substances that make us fat, sick, and unhappy, zapping our body of the necessary strength and energy needed to overcome our daily challenges. The healthier your overall diet becomes, the stronger and wiser your taste buds become. It takes time to retrain your brain and taste buds. I've found that when you detox the junk out of your diet, the cravings subside and your palate can heal. The good news is that our bodies are naturally inclined to find satisfaction in foods that sustain life and make us healthy. Find pleasure in the foods that nourish you. And if you haven't found them yet, keep looking. They do exist.

Admittedly, change can be difficult, and new foods don't always taste good on the first bite. So, keep this question in mind: Do I consistently find pleasure in my healthy food choices? If yes, chances for long-term success are excellent. If no, there is still work to do. Setbacks are normal; when you feel your motivation to keep eating well weaken, go back to your positive mind-set and press the reset button. With the proper mind-set, your OptimalBody approach to nutrition becomes clearer.

After reading this chapter, I hope you have a better understanding of how inflammation affects your body, the steps you can take to reduce it and balance the health of your gut, and the tools and mind-sets needed to stick with these changes. Because MS therapy is not associated with any official prescription for diet and lifestyle, we have to take personal responsibility to find the combination that works best for us. But one thing is certain: MS is an inflammatory disease, and MS symptoms can be made better when you control inflammation and the health of your gut. Remember, you're either fueling the fire or you're putting it out.

THE MULTI-PHASE
PLAN
TO
ACHIEVE
YOUR
OPTIMAL
BODY

CHAPTER 4

Getting Started
Know the Terms and Tools

When Darren and I developed the OptimalBody program, we knew the key was going to be a strong foundation—one you could build from and adapt. The foundation of this program is Phase 1.

Although it may, at first, look basic, Phase 1 is the most important phase of the program. You may face one or many limitations or challenges that can greatly affect your strength and mobility. For that reason, start with a basic strength-building phase to overcome those challenges—and to get you moving from Day 1, even if you've never worked out before. Also remember that the program is adaptable for any fitness level. We offer regressions of the movements (to make them easier) to allow anyone following the program the opportunity to find his or her individual starting point.

We also offer movement progressions (to make them harder). Some people will make tremendous progress against their limitations and be physically able to move on to the higher intensity of Phase 2. For these people, it is important to offer the later phases and not restrict their potential progress. Others will not make the type of progress that will allow them to move into these phases. The human body has a natural ability to adapt to stress; exercise is simply a form of physical stress used to make the muscles stronger. This is why it's important to know how you can take it to the next level—smartly and safely.

Darren and I know that multiple sclerosis offers many different challenges on a daily basis and that the program had to be designed with those challenges in mind. During my own early stages of training, we developed many of the adaptations needed to move forward. Adaptations may include alternate exercises with shortened ranges of motion to avoid muscle tears, placing the focus of the movement more on the contraction of the muscles rather than the stretch, and so on. This program is a direct result of my personal journey and challenges. Know we are in this together.

> The human body has a natural ability to adapt to stress; exercise is simply a form of physical stress used to make the muscles stronger.

It is impossible to address every limitation a person might confront, but we've made the program as complete and adaptable for as many people as possible to use it to regain control of their health and improve their quality of life. Whether facing a physical limitation, a debilitating disease, or any other challenge, this program creates an opportunity for people to assess the extent of their limitations and, perhaps, discover they aren't as limited as originally thought. The human body was designed to move. Movement is what keeps us healthy. Our goal is to get as many people moving as we possibly can.

With that said, let me issue a warning. When striving for certain goals, especially fitness-related goals, there will be obstacles. Remember they are just that—obstacles, not roadblocks. With determination and knowledge, any obstacle can be overcome. Education, along with an unwavering desire to succeed, can make a person unstoppable. With hard work and the right plan in place, which includes keeping safety foremost in mind, any goal is attainable. If an obstacle seems insurmountable, take the time to learn what else is possible, proceed with caution, and never give up.

With determination and knowledge, any obstacle can be overcome.

Our program has been tested and proven. Through the years, we have learned it's all about attitude, mind-set, and commitment. If we believe we are the best, we will become our best. We keep moving forward, stopping only long enough to learn and explore new ideas. You are now an OptimalBody athlete despite the hardships in your path. I believe in the Optimal-Body program, and I believe in you!

In this chapter, you will learn about the OptimalBody approach to training. The goal is to introduce you to a training system proven effective for people with health, physical, or emotional challenges. However, it is also adaptable for people with advanced fitness goals. Though there may be many effective forms of training out there, the OptimalBody approach is different. Your typical fitness program, advertised in infomercials or described in magazines, assumes the person performing the workout has no limitations.

The OptimalBody program understands everyone has a different starting point and that exercises may have to be modified depending on how you feel on any given day. What if you suffer from multiple sclerosis and experience symptoms of fatigue or neuropathy? Have COPD and lose your breath

 Doctor's Note

Once a goal is established with careful consideration of baseline capabilities in collaboration with a doctor, physical therapist, and trainer, working hard to achieve a goal like this is very possible for people with MS. As long as safety is addressed, most medical professionals would support a planned exercise routine.

easily? Were diagnosed with cancer and are recovering from chemotherapy? How do you jump into a regular exercise program to build strength and regain your health? If the program is not adaptable to an individual's fitness level, it will not work. It needs to be adjustable to a point where any person can have the confidence to begin, knowing they can work at their own pace and from a starting point that is safe for them. This is the basic concept of the OptimalBody approach to training.

The training is effective in that it combines the muscle-building component of resistance training with the fat-burning effects of cardio—all in one workout. It is an efficient way to reach your goals in a short amount of time without hours in the gym. The key to success is to find the right starting point and understand how to progress at a safe pace. There are a few essentials to keep in mind before you begin:

- **Get a complete physical evaluation from your doctor.** Get your doctor's input, concerns, and recommendations before you begin a new fitness program.
- **Work with a physical therapist** for rehabilitation and management of possible limitations.

- **Work with an exercise trainer** to help guide you through your exercise plans.
- **Understand your limitations and know the possible results** of trying to do too much too fast.
- **Listen to your body.** Be smart and know when to stop. Never lose sight of your goals, but never sacrifice health and safety while trying to reach them. Your body will tell you when enough is enough.

When it comes to health and fitness, there are no shortcuts to success. No magic formulas can replace hard work and proper nutrition. A lack of results is simply a matter of following the wrong path. You deserve to get the results you desire. It is my goal to provide you with a plan for success.

The human body has a remarkable ability to go into survival mode and adapt to physical stress. It is this ability that allows us to regain our health and well-being through physical exercise. It is of utmost importance when training to understand this and know how to press on and achieve your fitness goals. Having a simple understanding of how the body responds to training is important before proceeding. Please read this information carefully. If you have previous exercise experience, use this section to review the basics. Remember, the limitations that brought you to this program may require a different approach than you may be used to. A good foundation and understanding of the fundamentals are important when trying to attain a goal.

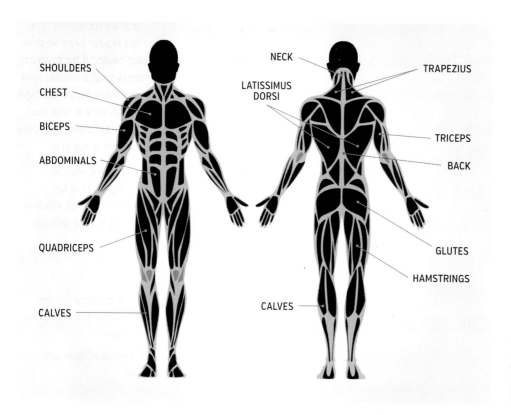

NECK
TRAPEZIUS
SHOULDERS
CHEST
LATISSIMUS DORSI
BICEPS
TRICEPS
ABDOMINALS
BACK
QUADRICEPS
GLUTES
HAMSTRINGS
CALVES
CALVES

The exercises in this book will work the muscles labeled in this diagram, alternating the focus between upper and lower body exercises.

BASIC OPTIMALBODY TERMINOLOGY

Before we move on, I will briefly explain what certain terms mean to make it easier to understand each exercise.

Repetition (rep): One sequence of a particular movement from the start position to the finish position. A normal repetition should be performed with a tempo (the speed of movement to complete the repetition) of 2–1–2. Simply stated, this means:

- Two seconds to perform the movement from the start position to the finish position

- A one-second pause to contract the working muscle

- Another two seconds to return to the starting position and be ready for the next repetition

Set: A group of consecutive repetitions to complete the exercise before moving on to the next set or next exercise. Rest time between sets in this program should be about forty-five seconds, unless otherwise specified. If an exercise is listed as 3 x 12 to 15, the athlete will perform three sets, each with twelve to fifteen repetitions of the exercise.

> Never sacrifice form and technique for a higher weight. You will only increase your risk of injury.

Note: Twelve to fifteen is the range of repetitions to be completed. If you can perform fifteen repetitions of the exercise on all three sets with good form, you will need to increase your working weight to challenge your muscle. If you cannot perform at least twelve repetitions on the last set of the exercise with good form, most likely you will need to decrease the working weight. Never sacrifice form and technique for a higher weight because you will only increase your risk of injury.

 Doctor's Note

Fatigue may make it harder to predict how many reps you can do. Always lowball the weight you use to allow enough repetitions.

Adaptation: Your body will try to adapt to any stress you put on it. In other words, it will fight you every step of the way to stay exactly the same as it is right now when you try to change your level of physical fitness. Your body does *not* want to change. You will have to make that change happen. How many times have you started a fitness program and been happy with the progress you were making, only to see that progress come to a screeching halt after a short period of time? While frustrating, this is simply a sign that something needs to be changed to start progressing again. This is even more important when dealing with limitations. In general, to regain strength, range of motion, or health, you must progress your workouts.

I stress again that this is done on an individual basis determined only by your own abilities, at your own pace. Do not worry if someone progresses faster than you. It is not important. What is important is that *you* are always making progress. The OptimalBody's approach to training—a twofold method using both resistance training and cardiovascular conditioning—is designed to overcome your body's attempts to adapt by stressing it in several different aspects at the same time, and making changes to keep you from getting stuck at a plateau. Learn more about how to adapt your workout on page 60.

Doctor's Note

Osteopenia (decreased bone density) and osteoporosis are common in MS, especially for those who have used steroids to treat the condition.

> In general, to regain strength, range of motion, or health, you must progress your workouts.

Resistance training: Resistance training means challenging the action of the muscles against an opposing force, such as a stationary object, manual resistance from a training partner, or weights. This is where it all happens. Resistance training has many health benefits, including increased strength, which helps you avoid muscle loss or atrophy, and it delays a decrease in bone density that occurs due to aging, lack of use, or certain conditions, such as osteoporosis.

Too many times people begin an exercise program that includes cardiovascular training without enough resistance training. But resistance training, or weight training, is where we build muscle to regain strength to perform activities for daily living (ADLs). It is also where we stimulate the body's metabolism, the rate at which we burn fat. A person's metabolism can be altered with changes in activity and proper nutrition habits. An inactive person tends to lose muscle, and that slows his or her metabolism. People who eat only once or twice a day will slow their metabolism by putting their bodies into starvation mode. In this condition, the body tries to burn

the calories from those meals more slowly to provide the body with enough energy to function throughout the day. A slow metabolism will cause a person to store calories as fat, while a fast metabolism will cause calories to be burned as fuel and keep them lean and healthy.

Muscle is the body's primary fat-burner. Sometimes, however, women hesitate to do weight training for fear of bulking up or looking like a man or a female bodybuilder. Remember, this program is called OptimalBody, and some female bodybuilders you see in magazines are anything but natural, and therefore by our definition, not optimal!

At OptimalBody, we do not condone or promote the use of performance-enhancing drugs. Even with the help of performance-enhancing drugs, it takes a lot of hard work to build the kind of muscle that will land you on the pages of a bodybuilding magazine. It doesn't happen by accident. The truth is, muscle is much denser than body fat, so 1 lb (455 g) of muscle will take up a lot less space than 1 lb (455 g) of body fat. With proper training and nutrition, you won't bulk up. Instead, you will achieve a body you can be proud of.

In traditional resistance training, exercises are broken up into sets and reps with rest periods between. For example, a person doing a biceps curl might perform the movement

8 to 10 times (reps) and then rest. Grouped together, these 8 to 10 reps make up a set. After the rest period, the person might perform several other groups of 8 to 10 repetitions, or additional sets. Those who want to build muscular strength generally do fewer reps with heavier weight (working the fast-twitch muscle fibers), while those who want to develop muscular endurance do higher reps with lighter weight (working the slow-twitch muscle fibers). The rest periods are usually longer when working with heavy weight and shorter when using light weight. The OptimalBody program uses a combination of different set and rep schemes to vary the stresses on the muscles, which works both types of muscle fibers. The more completely we stress a muscle, the more completely it has to rebuild and repair, leaner, stronger, and healthier.

Cardiovascular conditioning: Although muscle is the body's primary fat burner, cardiovascular training (or, simply, cardio) burns fat in other ways. It is a training method designed to raise a person's heart rate and burn more calories, as well as train the heart muscle to become stronger and work more efficiently. I recommend starting slowly. Again, how slow depends on your personal fitness level and limitations. Some people may start out with thirty minutes on a treadmill while others might start out with five minutes or fewer. Start at a place you can handle and increase gradually.

 Doctor's Note

A directed and consistent exercise plan may also have additional benefits, including lessening of fatigue, pain, cognitive problems, and imbalance, among other issues.

 Doctor's Note

For people with decreased mobility from MS, increased body weight is a risk. This can, in turn, impede mobility and exercise capability even more.

When losing weight is a major factor in your ability to regain health, the key is to create a deficit in which you burn more calories than you take in during the day. Cardiovascular training can help achieve that deficit and lead to the desired weight loss. Weight loss can have a broad range of benefits, from alleviating symptoms to allowing an individual to change or drop certain medications (in consultation with a physician).

When just beginning, many people ask if it is more important to start a workout with resistance training or cardiovascular training. One without the other creates a workout that is unbalanced and produces few results. In fact, cardiovascular training without resistance training often leads to muscle loss and can significantly slow a person's metabolism. The OptimalBody program combines the benefits of both types of training in a complete and efficient workout.

> Cardiovascular training without resistance training often leads to muscle loss and can significantly slow a person's metabolism. Both cardio and resistance training are needed for a complete and efficient workout.

Hypertrophic definition (HD): The OptimalBody program uses hypertrophic definition (HD) training. *Hypertrophy* is the physiological name for muscle growth, and *definition* refers to the training's cardiovascular aspect to help get lean. Thus, *hypertrophic definition* simply means performing muscle-building exercises with an elevated heart rate to burn calories and fat. The idea of the OptimalBody HD Training System is simple: You can build muscle and burn fat at the same time.

Circuit training: Circuit training is a method that involves grouping exercises together in such a way that you move quickly from one exercise to the next with little or no rest in between. This keeps the heart rate up and in an effective calorie-burning mode. Whether you want that beach body, to look like your favorite celebrity, or just need to combat specific symptoms, such as fatigue, this is an effective way to do it.

Mini circuits: These are small circuits grouped together to form a larger circuit. The OptimalBody program incorporates mini circuits in a variety of exercises to keep the workout fun and avoid overtraining on any particular movement.

Supersets: While circuits combine groups of exercises (usually four or more), supersets focus specifically on two exercises performed back to back with little or no rest in between before moving on to another exercise or another superset combining two more exercises.

HOW TO ADAPT FOR PROGRESSION OR MODIFY FOR REGRESSION

People face many kinds of limitations, and it is impossible to address them all. However, this section provides important information and guidelines on how to adapt the program to your specific needs. The program, as written, is designed to take you to a high level of fitness and intensity–but only if that is your goal. It is important to provide a higher level of training for people who are capable or wish to achieve an advanced level of fitness.

However, you may not have the desire for a high level of intensity, or you may have a limitation that will not currently allow you to train in this manner. It is important to understand that each phase in the program is a progression of the previous phase and should only be attempted if, and when, you are able to advance your training. In other words, some people–such as those simply looking to be more active–may never move on from Phase 1. That's okay! The basic strength-building effects of Phase 1 are sometimes all that are needed to live a more active and productive life. If that's the case for you, we also provide several ways to progress Phase 1 of the program, so while you continue to train in this phase you can improve and escalate results at your own pace. Following are some options for adapting this program to your specific needs and limitations.

> Some people–such as those simply looking to be more active–may never move on from Phase 1. That's okay!

Option 1:
Increase Reps for Muscular Endurance

To take Phase 1 to the next step, restart it and change the rep range to twenty to thirty reps to increase muscular endurance. Following this model, the repetitions could later be modified to an even higher range–fifty to one hundred–depending on ability and desired intensity level. We recommend that, at this high level of intensity, you cut the number of sets of each exercise to one or two to avoid overtraining.

Option 2:
Decrease Reps for Strength Building

Start Phase 1 again with fewer reps, such as five to eight, to shift the focus toward building strength. The program could also be modified on a weekly basis, completing one week with all exercises performed in a low-rep range (five to ten repetitions), followed by a week where the exercises are performed in a high-rep range (twenty to thirty repetitions). Or you might choose a 3-week cycle during which the rep range changes from low to medium to high, spending one week in each range (e.g., Week 1: perform all exercises with a rep range of five to ten; Week 2: perform all exercise with a rep range of twelve to fifteen; Week 3: perform all exercise with a rep range of twenty to thirty, and then start the cycle again with a week of low repetitions).

Option 3:
Perform a Circuit to Elevate Heart Rate

Phase 1 can also be modified to be performed in a circuit format to add variety. Perform one set of each exercise in Phase 1 and move to the next with little or no rest in between. This helps keep the heart rate elevated.

Option 4:
Use Supersets to Train Primary and Secondary Muscles Together

Repeat Phase 1 using supersets, pairing an exercise working a large muscle group, such as chest or back, with an exercise working a smaller muscle group, such as triceps or biceps, moving immediately from one to the other with no rest in between. On Day 2 of the program (legs), pair exercises for opposing muscle groups, such as quadriceps (the large muscles making up the front of the thighs) and hamstrings (the muscles making up the back of the thighs). Opposing muscles work against one another to allow side to side or up and down movement. For example, the biceps and triceps allow us to bend or straighten our lower arms by relaxing and contracting muscles in opposition to one another. So, for the legs, you may choose to do superset leg extensions (page 94) with seated leg curls (page 100) or leg presses (page 97) with stiff leg dead lifts (page 102).

Modifying Exercises

Within each phase, every exercise can be modified. Besides just adding more weight to the movements, there are progressions of the movement (making it harder) when an exercise becomes easy, and there are also regressions (making it easier) for when it is too difficult. Let's use a stationary lunge as an example.

Stationary Lunge

1. Stand with your feet in a lunge position, one foot stepped forward in front of the other while maintaining a shoulder-width distance between the feet for balance. Your feet should not be in line with one foot directly in front of the other. Your front foot will be flat on the floor, while your back foot will be up on the ball of your foot.

2. While holding onto something for support, bend both knees and lower your hips straight down. Your back knee should come down to where it lightly touches the floor while simultaneously bending your front knee to a 90-degree angle with your knee directly over your ankle.

3. To complete the repetition, extend both knees and raise your hips straight up, back to the starting position.

Now, you have several options for modifying the stationary lunge:

Progressions

- Add weight, such as holding dumbbells, a fixed-weight barbell, or bar, balanced across the upper back and shoulders.
- Make it a walking lunge by stepping forward or backward with each repetition.
- Perform the movement with either the front or back foot elevated to isolate the muscles further and challenge your balance and core strength.

But what do you do if performing a basic stationary lunge is too difficult? Simple, regress the movement until you achieve a level that can be performed safely.

Regressions

- If you struggle with balance, coordination, or leg strength, perform the stationary lunge in place where you can hold onto a wall, bar, or partner for balance.
- Perform a step-up or step-down onto a step or box with one foot, keeping the other foot planted, or step up or down with both feet. Hold onto a wall, bar, or partner for balance, if needed. The step-up or -down works the same muscles as the lunge but provides more stability and lower intensity.

Note that adding weight during progression is an individual adaptation that depends on your strength. The key is to use a slightly higher weight without jumping up too drastically in each progression.

The point is to find a version of each exercise you are comfortable to start with and gradually progress from there. Remember, simply going from a supported movement where you hold onto something for balance to an unsupported variation where you are able to let go is a progression. Small progress is still progress! Progress your movements at a rate comfortable and safe for you, especially if you are working without the help of a training partner or a professional trainer. If you do work with a partner, be sure he fully understands your limitations. Also, be patient with your progress. Don't be afraid to challenge yourself, but always do so in a controlled and safe way to avoid injury. Many injuries occur when we get impatient and try to accomplish too much too quickly.

Small progress is still progress!

Another way to modify your exercise is with time. It does not matter how long you spend in each phase of this program. You may spend as much time as you need in any phase, or you may never progress to the next phase. Your goals and abilities determine how you move through the different phases. Make sure the goals you set are reasonable and attainable. A person recovering from a stroke or with a debilitating illness should not approach the training with the intention of becoming the next Mr. Universe, but should look at Phase 1 as a way to regain strength, health, and independence, or as a supplement to physical therapy.

Each day of the program is adaptable, as well. If Day 1 is too intense as written, simply cut back on the volume of training. You can cut back on the number of exercises for each muscle group, or the number of sets performed for each exercise. If the program calls for 3 chest exercises, but you can only do 1, then start there and add a second one when you get a little stronger. This is a lifelong journey of health and fitness, not a mad dash to some imaginary finish line. Challenge yourself but work at your own pace and keep safety as the number one priority.

To provide an example for an upper body movement, any of the chest exercises can be progressed or regressed, as well.

Progressions	Regressions
Add weight to challenge the muscle further.	Perform a push-up using only your body weight.
Shorten the range of motion to perform partial repetitions (press the weight only half way up off the chest and don't lock the arms out before lowering the weight back to the chest) to eliminate the help from the triceps in locking out the arms at full extension, thereby keeping the tension strictly on the chest muscles instead.	Perform a modified push-up with knees bent, touching the floor, rather than a regular push-up with knees straight and toes on the floor.
	Perform a hand-release push-up by lowering your body all the way down until you are lying flat on the floor. Raise your hands off the floor by your shoulders (in push-up position) and then, with a thrusting motion, put your hands back on the floor and "push through" as if you were pushing the floor away from your body. The hand-release push-up does not require you to balance your body weight off the floor.
	Reduce the angle of your body in a regular push-up to reduce resistance. Perform a push-up with your hands on a bench, countertop, or against the adjustable height of the bar in a Smith Machine (see page 65). You can even place your hands against a wall and push away instead of pushing up.

How Much Weight Should I Lift?

When beginning any exercise program, the amount of weight used in each set is important. You want to perform every set to a failure point at the final rep instructed for each movement. In other words, you want to try, if possible, to increase the weight load as you decrease the reps set by set. The more you demand of your muscles without overtraining, the better the results you will achieve.

Remember: Safety, proper form, and focus always come first while exercising. When working with a personal trainer, he or she will be instrumental in determining the amount of weight to use. When working out on your own, it will take a little more time and several workouts to find the proper amount. Be patient and know it will take some trial and error to discover the correct weights for you. This is a lifestyle, not a quick fix for your health. You have a lifetime ahead of you!

I can't stress enough the importance of keeping good form on all exercises. You should never sacrifice form to use a heavier weight. The only thing you will accomplish is increasing your risk of injury. You can't expect to reach your goals if you're sitting at home injured. Always train smart; never ego lift. The quality of the movement is more important than how much weight you're using.

Avoid Overtraining

The OptimalBody HD Training System recognizes that you need to avoid overtraining to keep results coming. Overtraining can be simply using too much weight or not allowing enough rest and recovery time for a specific muscle group. In either case, you are only decreasing your potential for results while increasing your potential risk for injury. Due to the high intensity of the OptimalBody HD Training System, it is possible to overtrain if you are not properly conditioned. Varying the intensity can help prevent overtraining, as well as accommodate limitations.

We also recommend a variety of training styles to avoid getting stuck at a plateau. We've found that some people can avoid plateaus and achieve great results by alternating weeks of the program with weeks of a more traditional training style. For example, during Phase 2, you can perform the exercises as written with the Metabolism Jump Starts (page 121) between each set. After a week (or several weeks) you may choose to lower the intensity, allowing the body some rest time, and omit these movements between sets, simply performing the exercises as written. This would lower the intensity to something comparable to Phase 1 for a short time before picking it back up. During this time, you could incorporate other techniques, such as:

- Negatives (lowering the weight at a much slower than normal speed to keep tension on the working muscles for an extended period of time)
- Partial reps (performing the repetitions through a shortened range of motion when the muscle becomes tired)
- Drop sets (performing a certain number of repetitions and then reducing the weight to perform additional repetitions)

Remember, the OptimalBody HD Training System is adaptable to many different fitness levels, on an individual and as-needed basis.

ADAPTING PHASE 1 SPECIFICALLY TO YOU

When adapting a fitness program, you have to consider fitness level, overall health, limitations, and goals—but MS adds another complication. As a person with a disability, I know there is no easy way to dive into a workout routine. But the fact is, working out is not an option but a necessity in overcoming the challenge you face.

The first thing I did when I got back into the gym was to assess the damage, so to speak. MS has left me with nerve damage from the attack that led to my diagnosis, a common symptom among MS sufferers. Whether you are battling MS or another degenerative condition, there are physical symptoms and limitations you must take into consideration before you begin a workout program.

Grip and Numbness

MS affects my left side considerably more than my right. My left hand does not close easily, my grip is impaired, and my hand goes numb. With these concerns, some exercises are problematic and may even cause an injury if I don't address the symptoms and adapt the movement. To compensate for these issues, I do not perform any dumbbell movements that place the dumbbells above my head or face, or in any position that would injure me if one fell. Instead, I adapt the exercises to use weight-stacked machines, weighted cable movements, or non-weighted resistance bands. I recommend the same for people with MS who have trouble holding free weights in either hand due to weakness, incoordination, or similar problems.

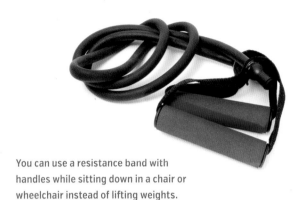

You can use a resistance band with handles while sitting down in a chair or wheelchair instead of lifting weights.

Resistance bands (I recommend the ones with handles) can help you perform the same movement you would perform with free weights, dumbbells, fixed-weight barbells, bars (with or without weight plates), or machines. The challenge is creating enough resistance; a shorter band or one with more tension offers stronger resistance. Weightlifting straps are another way to help you overcome the challenges with grip or feeling in the hands and fingers. The straps allow weight to be lifted by transferring the load to the wrists and avoiding limitations in fingers, the hand, or grip strength.

Balance

Balance is another issue that plagues MS sufferers. In standing movements, such as squats or lunges, you can use the Smith machine, which balances the exercise for you. Personally, I live under a Smith machine while at the gym and perform many of my movements using it.

Know your limits every time you walk into a gym, with or without a trainer. Find ways to steady yourself and secure yourself while working out. And while moving from machine to machine, do not be afraid or embarrassed to hold onto the wall, the equipment, or your trainer. You are a champion and should be proud of your accomplishment of being in the gym while many are sitting on couches doing nothing to stay fit. Adapt your workout to guarantee it is safe and effective.

Following are the exercises for Phase 1 of the OptimalBody HD Training System, with alternate means to execute them to adapt to your condition or challenge.

A Smith machine is designed to balance your body and help you control the weights no matter your condition. This weight machine consists of a bar (with or without weight plates) that slides on a fixed rail, and can lock into place at the fixed points along the track. Twisting the bar activates J-shaped hooks on its side that lock into holes on the rails. This simple locking mechanism makes it easier to work on exercises, such as squats, bench presses, and shoulder presses, whether you're with your trainer or alone at the gym, effectively turning the Smith machine into a spotter. This is a perfect machine for those of us who have problems with balance, difficulty gripping, or numbness.

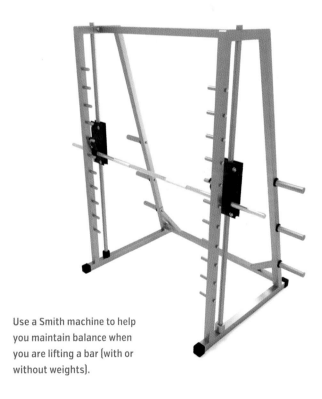

Use a Smith machine to help you maintain balance when you are lifting a bar (with or without weights).

Adapting in a Wheelchair

Even though it is challenging to train with MS, it is even more of an effort when you are in a wheelchair with MS. I am here to tell those of you in wheelchairs, you can do it! There are many upper body exercises that can be done from a wheelchair with weights and exercise bands. I'm going to outline some exercises from Phase 1 using resistance bands.

This is a beginner routine, and more exercises can be added once you are comfortable. The key is to start somewhere. It's important, especially with MS from a wheelchair, to keep the body moving and stay active. You have to stay motivated and never quit!

Resistance bands can be purchased with different levels of resistance and typically come in a package, allowing you to increase the resistance as your strength increases. Follow the same OptimalBody HD Training System guidelines for sets and repetitions, but use the bands while sitting in your wheelchair. Simple, right?! Make sure you exhale on exertion and inhale at release. Always sit tall in your chair, and keep your abdominals tight.

OPTIMALBODY TRAINING STEP BY STEP

Let's take a closer look at the structure of the OptimalBody approach to training. We must train the entire body to achieve maximum results and avoid muscle imbalances that could lead to injury. If you have a limitation that affects the strength of a particular muscle group, you still need to dedicate time to training these weaker muscles rather than just focusing on your strengths. For example, if you're dependent on a walker for mobility, you still want to train your leg muscles to try to regain some strength and flexibility. Some exercises might need to be modified, and some movements might need to be regressed. By combining a balance of strength training with cardiovascular conditioning, the OptimalBody approach helps you build muscle while simultaneously keeping the heart strong and reducing body fat to avoid potential health risks associated with higher body fat percentages. Of course, proper nutrition is required to make it all effective.

In Phase 1 of the OptimalBody program, we recommend starting with a traditional type of cardiovascular training, such as using a treadmill, stair climber, elliptical glider, exercise bike, or hand bike, for twenty minutes. This, of course, depends on your physical abilities and inclinations. You may need to start with ten minutes or fewer if twenty is just too much. As always, keep safety foremost in your mind. At the beginning, go with the amount of time that pushes you a bit beyond your comfort zone without overdoing it. Also, choose a cardiovascular machine or exercise that works within your limitations. I can no longer use an elliptical glider due to lack of coordination in my left leg, but I can manage a treadmill or bike without the same difficulty. Remember that working out may not be an easy task, but fitness can and should be a combination of fun and results.

Later, as your cardiovascular conditioning improves, the exercises in Phase 1 can be performed in a circuit format. To perform a circuit, perform 1 set of each exercise and move to the next with little or no rest in between. This helps keep the heart rate elevated. After completing 1 set of each prescribed exercise for the particular day, you would then take a short rest and start again, performing a second set of each exercise. Repeat for a third set of each exercise.

You will notice that on Day 1 all exercises are performed for three sets. This makes for an easy transition to the circuit format. On Days 2 and 3, however, some exercises are performed for only three or four sets. In this case, you have options: Perform three sets of each exercise and drop any exercises with only two sets [e.g., assisted pull-up [page 108] and straight-arm lat pulldown [page 115] on Day 3] from the third circuit, completing the last circuit with only the remaining exercises; or finish the exercises with more than three sets at the end of the circuit to complete all prescribed sets [as with squats on Day 2 [page 96]].

While both phases of the OptimalBody HD Training System incorporate a cardiovascular component, Phase 2 takes this to a higher intensity level. Learn to listen to your body and progress at a rate that keeps you safe and comfortable.

Phase 1 Sample Circuit

DAY 1

1. Perform first set of each exercise.
2. Short rest.
3. Perform second set of each exercise.
4. Short rest.
5. Perform third set of each exercise.

DAY 2

1. Perform first set of each exercise.
2. Short rest.
3. Perform second set of each exercise.
4. Short rest.
5. Perform third set of each exercise, skipping any exercises with only two sets.

DAY 3

1. Perform first set of each exercise.
2. Short rest.
3. Perform second set of each exercise.
4. Short rest.
5. Perform third set of each exercise, skipping any exercises with only two sets.
6. Short rest.
7. If desired, complete the fourth set of any four-set exercises.

CHAPTER 5

Phase 1
Adapt Your Workouts, Build Muscle, and Lose Fat

The goal in this approach, using the OptimalBody HD Training System, is to create and incorporate the positive aspects of a fitness program that is sustainable for a lifetime. It doesn't matter whether you are thirty or seventy years old when you start. What matters is you start today and move forward.

Phase 1 is a basic strength-building phase, the foundation of your exercise regimen. This phase focuses on hypertrophic definition–building muscle and losing fat. It is important to begin and continue with Phase 1 for a minimum of 2 to 4 weeks. During this time, you will have the opportunity to assess your progress and plan your future steps. If you're just starting your fitness journey, this is the most important phase of the program. This phase can be a standalone program for many of you. It may be all you need to regain the strength to perform your daily activities. This is the phase in which you will learn the basics, the foundation of exercises that will build strength, conditioning, and the confidence to continue.

Stretch
The fitness community has many opinions on the topic of stretching. Some people argue you should stretch before your workout, while others say you should stretch after. I have learned, through trial and error, there is no definitive answer on this. There are benefits to both.

Stretching after your first sets of a muscle group allows that muscle to become warmed up before the stretch. Why is this important? Stretching a cold muscle can possibly lead to a torn muscle or tendon, just as going into a workout without warming up can do the same. Once you finish this first stretching session, you can continue to train harder and with heavier weights while minimizing the chance of injury.

I have also seen, through more than thirty years of training, that stretching the muscles worked after the workout can help eliminate that tight, stiff feeling that seems to creep up on you a day or so later. The takeaway is to listen to your body in every workout. Concentrate on the stretch you are doing and do not overstretch the muscle. Extend the stretch to the point of feeling the muscle's elongation without going so far that you feel discomfort. At the beginning of your fitness journey, it's better to underperform than overperform. Stretching is an important part of your workout.

> ## At the beginning of your fitness journey, it's better to underperform than overperform.

Once you really know your body, you can push that stretch a bit farther. But remember, no matter your level, stretching cold or training without warming up can be disastrous. Because many of us with MS struggle with sensitivity in our limbs from neuropathy, tingling, and similar concerns, we should carefully perform every movement.

Warm-Up

As with any exercise program, spend a few minutes warming up your muscles to avoid injuries before jumping into your workout. Remember, you are making ZERO progress toward your goals if you are sitting at home injured!

A warm-up can be as simple as ten minutes on a treadmill, starting at a comfortable pace and gradually increasing to slightly more than comfortable. Don't go at a high intensity. This time should be spent just as a warm-up, not part of the workout. If you don't like, or want to avoid, the treadmill, you might use the elliptical machine or stationary bike. You can also do body weight exercises, such as jumping jacks or squats. People confined to wheelchairs may choose to use a hand bike. The point is to get the body moving and blood flowing to the muscles. A warm muscle will respond better and is less susceptible to injuries or tears.

Cardiovascular training (using a cardio machine) may be used as your warm-up. I prefer to warm up for ten minutes, get my weight training in, and then go back to a cardiovascular machine for another twenty minutes at the end of my workout. But this is your workout, not mine. There is no right or wrong way to get the cardiovascular section of your program accomplished. Find what you like, what works for you, and what fits into your schedule.

Once I begin my exercises, I usually do a few sets of the first exercise for each muscle group and perform the movements with light weights. This allows me to make my warm-up specific to the muscles I will be working and further reduces my risk of injury. The warm-up becomes even more important as we age, or if you are dealing with some sort of physical limitation that might make it easier to be injured.

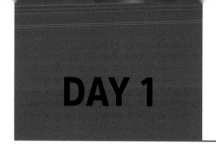

DAY 1

CHEST, SHOULDERS, TRICEPS, AND ABS

In Day 1, we will focus on the chest, shoulders, triceps, and abdominal muscles. The triceps muscles are worked on the same day as the chest muscles because they are the secondary muscles used in any chest movement. All exercises can be performed alone or with the aid of a spotter for safety, especially if you are just beginning or you experience symptoms in the muscles being worked, such as fatigue or spasticity.

Incline Bench Press

3 SETS — 1 each of 12 reps, 10 reps, and 8 reps

Equipment needed: incline bench with dumbbells or Smith machine with bar (with or without weight plates)

This exercise works your chest muscles with an emphasis on the upper chest. It also works the shoulders and triceps while lifting either a bar (supported by the Smith Machine) or dumbbells over your chest. You have a choice of which equipment you use and can alternate these as desired.

1 If using an adjustable bench, set the incline at approximately 30 degrees, which is the optimal angle to work the upper chest.

2 To start, grip the bar or dumbbells with a slightly wider-than-shoulder-width grip. The starting position should be across the upper chest.

3 Squeeze the muscles of your chest as you press the weight over your chest. If using dumbbells, bring the dumbbells together over your chest as you press upward.

4 With controlled movement, return the weight to the starting position to complete the repetition. Avoid letting the weight fall back to the starting position or bounce off your chest because this can cause injury.

Your Workout Week

Though this is the first day of the workout, it may not actually occur on the first day of your workout week. Because this program is based on a three-day workout schedule, you can easily adapt it for more days per week. For example, if you train four days per week, you will repeat Day 1 on Day 4 and begin the next week with Day 2 exercises.

Smith Machine Incline Bench Press

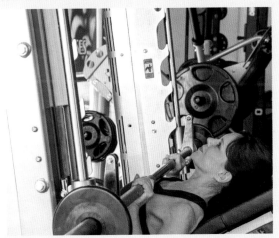
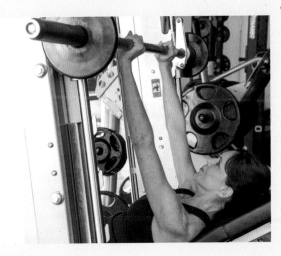

Incline Bench Press with Dumbbells

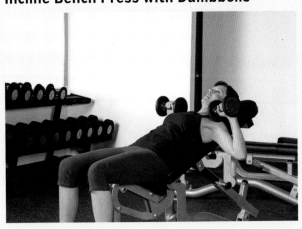
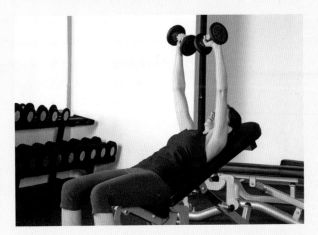

Machine Chest Press

3 SETS ▸ 1 each of 12 reps, 10 reps, and 8 reps

Equipment needed:
chest press machine

This exercise works your chest muscles, with an emphasis on your middle chest, as well as your shoulders and triceps, while you press the machine's handles forward in front of your body in an upright, seated position.

1 Sit in the machine and grip the handles at a height that is even with the middle of your chest and plant your feet firmly on the floor.

2 Squeeze the muscles of your chest as you press forward to full extension.

3 With controlled movement, return the weight to the starting position to complete each repetition.

 To Perform in a Wheelchair

1 Loop the resistance band around the back of the wheelchair and grasp the handles (one in each hand) at chest level, and back far enough so you are able to feel the resistance.

2 Press the bands forward until your arms are straight out in front of you. Do not lock your arms. You want to keep the tension throughout the movement, not relax in a locked position.

3 Slowly return to the starting position.

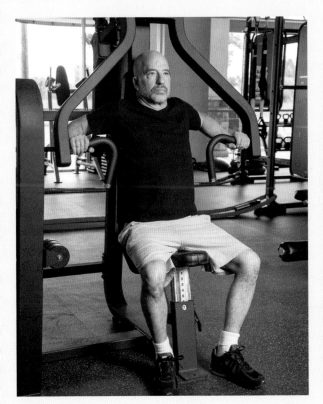 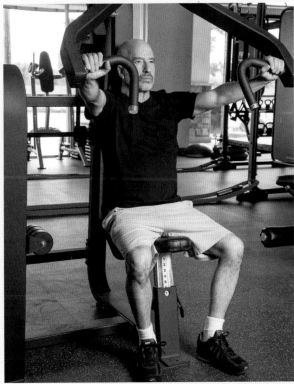

Phase 1: Day 1

Incline Dumbbell Fly or Cable Crossover

3 SETS 10 to 12 reps each

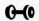 **Equipment needed:** incline bench with dumbbells or cable crossover machine

This exercise works your chest muscles, with an emphasis on your outer chest during the stretch position and the inner chest during the contracted position, as well as the shoulders, while starting in a wide, arms outstretched position and moving to a contracted position in front of the body. You have a choice of equipment and can alternate these as desired.

1 Set the bench position to a 30-degree angle, which is optimal. If using dumbbells, start with the dumbbells raised over your chest, with your palms facing each other and elbows slightly bent.

If using cables, stand with one foot forward for balance and grip the handles in the same position as you would the dumbbells.

2 To begin the repetition, open your arms wide and bend your elbows slightly more as you stretch your chest.

3 At the widest position, your elbows should be slightly bent to stretch your chest and your hands should not go past your shoulders to avoid injury.

4 Squeeze your chest as you continue through an arcing motion to a position back in front of your chest, with slightly less bend in your elbows, to complete the repetition.

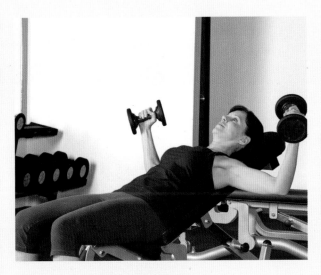

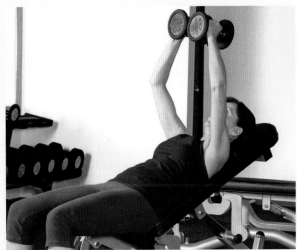

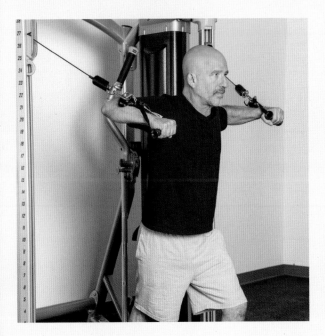

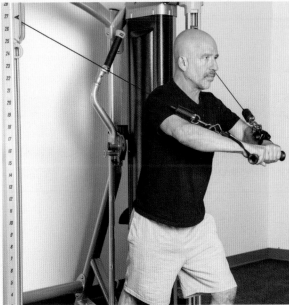

Dumbbell Shoulder Press

3 SETS 1 each of 12 reps, 10 reps, and 8 reps

Equipment needed: dumbbells

This exercise works your shoulder muscles and triceps while you raise the dumbbells overhead.

1 Start with the dumbbells at your shoulders, palms facing forward.

2 Press the dumbbells overhead and together.

3 To complete the repetition, return the dumbbells in a controlled movement to a position that is even with your earlobes. Don't go lower to avoid unnecessary stress on your shoulder joint.

To Perform a Shoulder Press in a Wheelchair

1 Secure the resistance band by looping it under the wheelchair's wheels.

2 Grasp the band handles and position them around your shoulder area. Keep your forearms straight and your hands at ear level.

3 Press the bands over your head. Your arms should extend just short of locking the elbows.

4 Slowly lower the bands back to the starting position and repeat the movement.

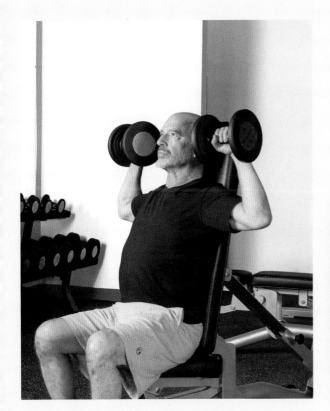 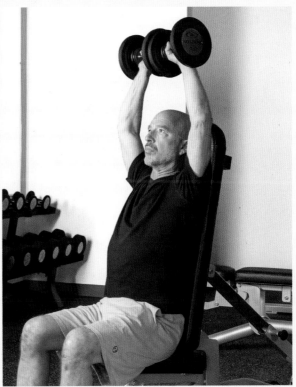

Dumbbell Lateral Raise

3 SETS   1 each of 8 reps,
10 reps, and 12 reps

Equipment needed:
dumbbells

This exercise works your shoulder muscles with an emphasis on the medial head while
you raise the dumbbells to the sides of your body.

1 Start with the dumbbells at your sides or in front
of your body with your palms facing inward and a
slight bend in your elbows.

2 Keeping the bend in your elbows consistent, lift
the dumbbells straight out to your sides and away
from your body to a position parallel to the floor.

3 Return the dumbbells to the starting position
in a controlled movement to complete the repetition.
Avoid swinging the weights to prevent injury.

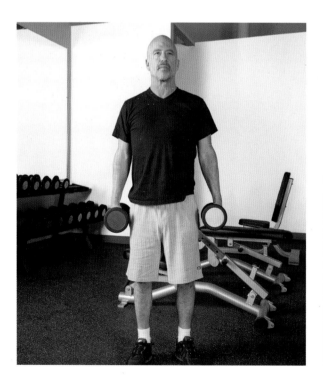
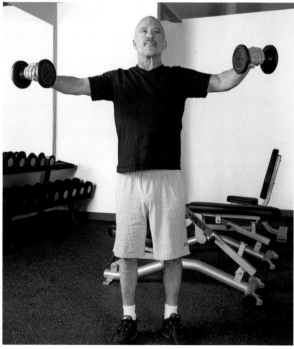

Dumbbell Front Raise

3 SETS — 10 to 12 reps each

Equipment needed: dumbbells

This exercise works your shoulder muscles, with an emphasis on the anterior head while you raise the dumbbells to the front of your body.

1 Start with the dumbbells in front of your body with your palms resting on your thighs and your elbows slightly bent to avoid stress on your joints.

2 Lift the dumbbells straight up in front of your body to eye level. This can be done simultaneously, or alternating.

3 With controlled movement, return the dumbbells to the starting position to complete the repetition. Avoid swinging the weights to prevent injury.

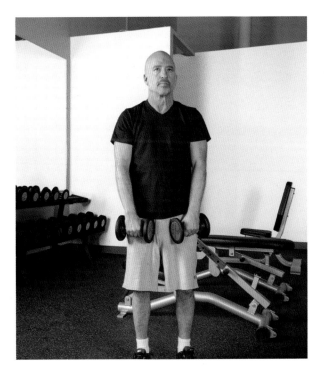
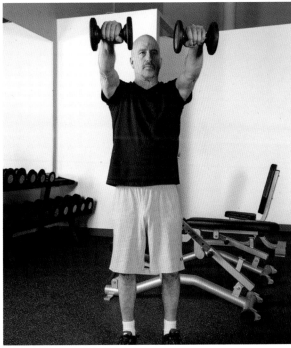

Bent-Over Dumbbell Lateral Raise

3 SETS   10 to 12 reps each

Equipment needed:
dumbbells and flat bench (optional)

This exercise works your shoulder muscles, with an emphasis on the posterior head. This is done while you raise the dumbbells out to the sides of your body in a bent-over position with your upper body parallel to the floor. This exercise can be performed either in a standing or seated position.

1 If performing the exercise standing, stand with your feet together and knees slightly bent. Keep your lower back tucked in to prevent injury and bend forward until your upper body is parallel to the floor.

2 Start with the dumbbells in front of your body, under your chest, with your palms facing each other and your elbows slightly bent.

If performing the exercise in a seated position, sit on the edge of the bench and lean forward with your chest on your thighs. Start with the dumbbells underneath your legs and palms facing together.

3 Keeping your upper body parallel to the floor and your elbows slightly bent, raise the dumbbells to the outside in an arcing motion. Keep your shoulders, elbows, and hands all in the same plane of movement.

4 With controlled movement, return the dumbbells to the starting position to complete the repetition.

To Perform a Reverse Fly in a Wheelchair

1 Fold your resistance band in half and grip each end in front of your chest, arms extended away from your body and elbows bent.

2 Pull the band apart, bringing it closer to your chest and straightening your arms and then slowly release it back to the start position.

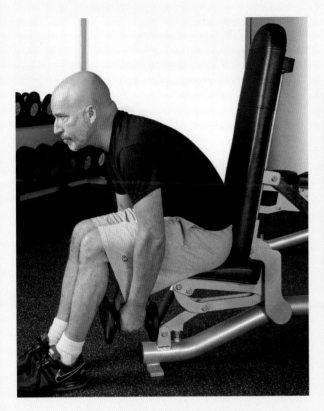 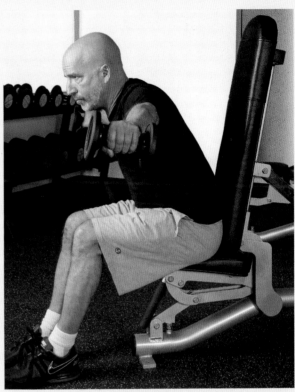

Lying Triceps Extension

3 SETS ⟩ 1 each of 12 reps, 10 reps, and 8 reps

Equipment needed: flat bench and fixed-weight barbell or E-Z curl bar (with or without weight plates)

This exercise works your triceps muscles while you lie flat on a bench, hold a bar over your chest, and bend your elbows to lower the bar toward your head.

1 Lie on a flat bench with your arms extended over your chest. Grip the bar at shoulder width.

2 Keeping your upper arm stationary, bend your arms at your elbow and, with controlled movement, lower the weight toward your forehead or hairline. Avoid contact with your forehead to prevent injury.

3 To complete the repetition, squeeze your triceps and raise the weight back to the starting position.

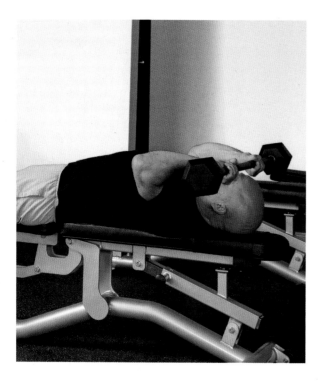
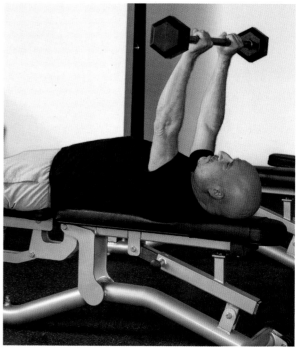

Triceps Dip

3 SETS 1 each of 12 reps, 10 reps, and 8 reps

 Equipment needed:
dip machine

The triceps dip is performed on a dip machine while pressing your arms to a fully extended position, raising your body.

1 Sit or stand in the machine with your back pressed firmly against the pad.

2 Grip the handles on the sides of the machine and squeeze your triceps muscles as you press downward to extend your arms fully.

3 With controlled movement, return to the starting position to complete the repetition.

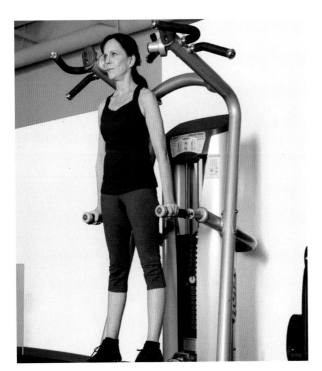
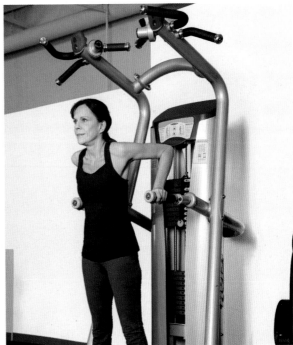

Triceps Pushdown

3 SETS 10 to 12 reps each

 Equipment needed: cable machine with pulley in the high position and straight bar or V-bar attachment

This exercise, using a high pulley cable machine, works your triceps muscles while you keep your elbows near your ribs and extend your arms in front of your body to a fully extended position.

1 Stand with your knees slightly bent and your feet together, or one foot slightly forward for balance. Grip the bar and keep your elbows on your ribs, close to your body.

2 Moving your arm from your elbow like a hinge, squeeze your triceps muscles and press the weight downward to a fully extended position.

3 To complete the repetition, keep your elbows at your ribs and return the weight to the starting position with your hands ending at chest level.

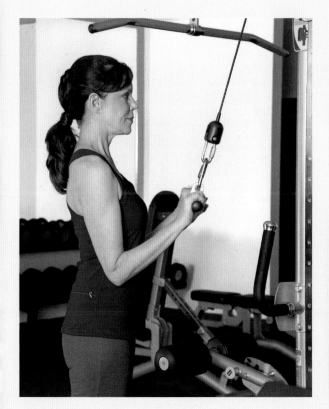
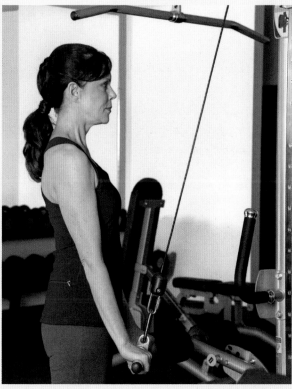

Overhead Cable Triceps Extension

3 SETS 10 to 12 reps each

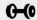 **Equipment needed:** cable machine with pulley in the low position and rope attachment

This exercise works your triceps muscles while you stand with your back to a cable machine and raise the weight overhead using a rope attachment connected to a low pulley.

1 Stand with your back to the cable machine, feet slightly wider than shoulder width and knees slightly bent for balance. Grip the ends of the rope attachment with your elbows high and your hands starting behind your head.

2 Keeping your upper arm stationary, squeeze your triceps and extend the cable to a fully overhead position.

3 With controlled movement, lower the weight to the starting position for a full stretch of your triceps to complete the repetition.

 ## To Perform an Overhead Triceps Extension in a Wheelchair

1 Secure the resistance band under the chair's wheels and grasp both handles of the bands and pull your arms close to the sides of your head, elbows pointing forward.

2 Extend your arms up, lifting the handles toward the ceiling, and then slowly release back to the starting position. The only movement should be your elbows bending and straightening. Keep your elbows pointed forward, not out to your sides.

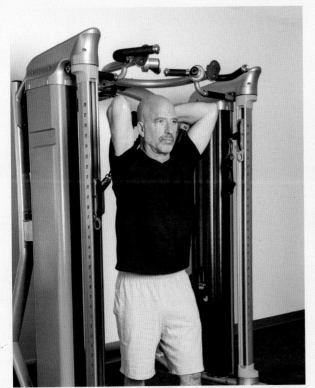 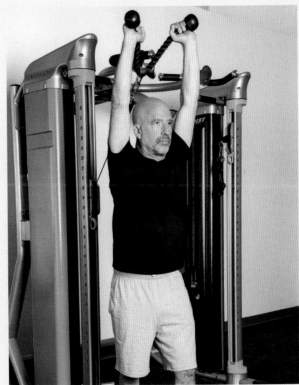

Leg Raise

3 SETS   20 to 25 reps each

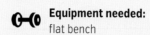 **Equipment needed:**
flat bench

For this exercise, you may choose to perform the leg raise, hip thrust (page 91), or knee tuck (page 90). Leg raises work the lower portion of the abdominal muscles while raising the legs from an extended position in front of your body to a position perpendicular to your upper body.

1 Lie flat on the bench and grip it on both sides of your head for stability. Start with your legs straight out and in line with your upper body.

2 Slowly contract your lower abdominal muscles as you raise your legs to 90 degrees. Avoid bending your knees.

3 To complete the repetition, slowly lower your legs to the starting position.

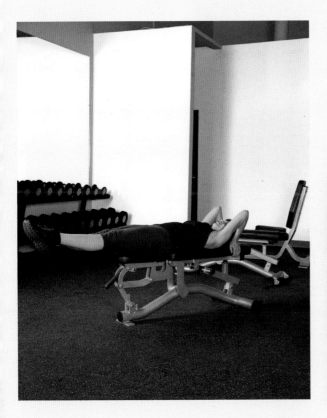
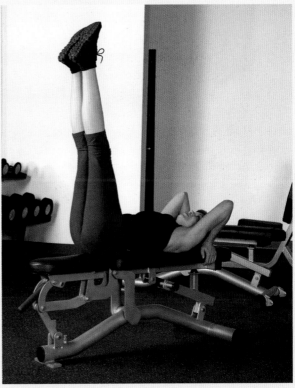

Knee Tuck

3 SETS   20 to 25 reps each

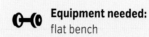 **Equipment needed:**
flat bench

Instead of the leg raise on page 88, you may choose to perform the knee tuck. Knee tucks work the lower portion of the abdominal muscles while sitting on the edge of a flat bench with your legs extended downward at a 45-degree angle and pulling your knees toward your chest.

1 Sit on the edge of the bench and lean slightly backward, with your legs extended downward at about a 45-degree angle, feet together. Grip the bench behind your hips for stability.

2 To perform the repetition, contract your abdominal muscles and bend your knees to pull your legs toward your chest while simultaneously bringing your upper body slightly forward.

3 Return to the starting position.

Online Exerise Images

To conserve space, some of the simpler exercises have been listed with descriptions only and do not include any photos. For people unfamiliar with these movements, we recommend the use of an online exercise library. One of the most complete that I have found is on www.BodyBuilding.com and can be accessed at www.bodybuilding.com/exercises/list/index/selected/a. Some of the exercises may have a slightly different name than what is listed in our program, but they can also be searched by muscle group on the same link by clicking on the tab at the top of the page.

Hip Thrust

3 SETS 20 to 25 reps each

 Equipment needed:
flat bench

Instead of the leg raise on page 88 or the knee tuck, opposite, you may choose to perform the hip thrust. Hip thrusts work the lower portion of your abdominal muscles while raising your hips off the bench and pushing your feet toward the ceiling.

1 Lie flat on the bench and grip it on both sides of your head for stability.

2 With your legs straight up and 90 degrees to your torso, contract your lower abdominal muscles as you push your feet toward the ceiling and raise your hips several inches (10 to 15 cm) off the bench.

3 Return to the starting position to complete the repetition.

To Perform a Seated Abs Stretch in a Wheelchair

1 Sit at the edge of your wheelchair.

2 Extend your legs out and your arms up overhead, stretching through the abs.

3 Hold for 10 to 30 seconds.

Crunch

3 SETS ▶ 20 to 25 reps each

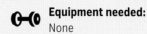 **Equipment needed:**
None

This exercise works your abdominal muscles while you lie on the floor and lift your shoulders to contract your muscles.

1 Lie flat on the floor with your knees bent and your feet flat on the floor. Place your hands loosely behind your head with your elbows pointing out to the sides.

2 To perform the repetition, contract your abdominal muscles and raise your shoulders off the floor while simultaneously pressing your lower back into the floor. Raise your chin straight up toward the ceiling and avoid pulling on your head to prevent neck injuries.

 To Perform a Seated Abs Crunch in a Wheelchair

1 Sit at the edge of your wheelchair.

2 With feet on the floor, slowly tighten your abdominal muscles "crunching" them forward. Do not lean your body forward more than slightly during the movement. The object is to compress the ab muscles, flexing them downward.

3 Release the crunch position and repeat for 20 reps. Your goal should be to do this routine 3 times per week on non-consecutive days.

Medicine Ball Russian Twist

3 SETS

20 to 25 reps each

Equipment needed:
medicine ball

This exercise works your abdominal and oblique muscles while you move a medicine ball from side to side across your body in a rotational movement.

1 Sit on the floor with your knees slightly bent and feet out in front, heels resting lightly on the floor or slightly off the floor for added difficulty. Your upper body should be angled back about 45 degrees. Grasp a medicine ball in front of your abdominal muscles.

2 To perform the repetition, rotate your upper body and touch the medicine ball to the floor on one side of your body while keeping your legs in a stationary position. Turn your head, not just your shoulders, and look at the ball to rotate your entire midsection.

3 Bring the medicine ball across your body and touch the floor on the opposite side of your body.

DAY 2

LEGS

On Day 2, we will focus on the leg muscles, the largest muscles of the body, which require a large amount of effort to work. For this reason, we've dedicated an entire day to them. Use a spotter for certain movements, such as squats and leg presses, because of the increased risk of injury while doing these movements alone.

Leg Extension

3 SETS ▶ 1 each of 12 reps, 10 reps, and 8 reps

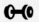 **Equipment needed:** leg extension machine

This exercise works your quadriceps muscles by extending your legs in front of your body.

1 Sit in the machine with your back placed firmly against the back pad and the lower pad on the front of your ankles. Your knee joint should be in alignment with the machine's pivot point.

2 Simultaneously raise your legs to their full extension.

3 Squeeze your quadriceps muscles at the top of the movement before lowering the weight, with controlled movement, back to the starting position to complete the repetition.

 To Perform a Seated Leg Extension in a Wheelchair

1 Secure your left foot in the resistance band's handle. Place the band under the right wheel, holding the remaining band in your right hand.

2 Sit tall without leaning back. Lift your left leg so the back of your thigh comes off the seat.

3 Extend the elevated leg straight and then bend it. The only movement should come from bending and extending your knee. Keep your left thigh lifted off your seat the entire time.

4 Repeat the exercise with your right foot in the band handle and the band under the left wheel.

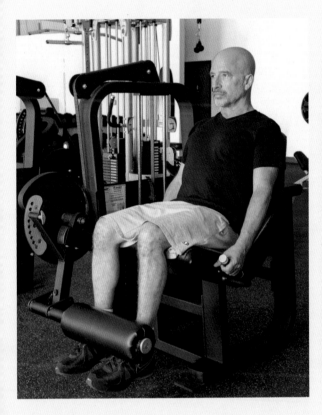 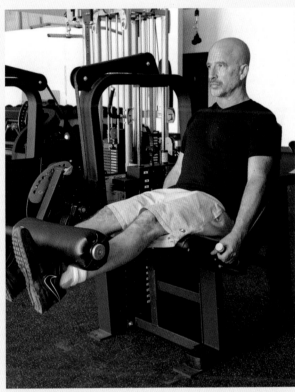

Squat

4 SETS 8 to 12 reps each

Equipment needed: squat rack and bar (with or without weight plates)

This exercise works your quadriceps, hamstrings, and gluteal muscles while you stand with a weight balanced across your upper back and shoulders and squat to a position where your hips are below your knees.

1 Start with the bar across your upper back and your feet shoulder width apart or slightly wider.

2 Keep your lower back tucked in and your chest up as you bend at the knees and hips to a full squat position, where your hips are slightly below the knee joint. Always align the knees with the toes to avoid injury.

3 Avoid leaning forward as you return to a standing position to complete the repetition.

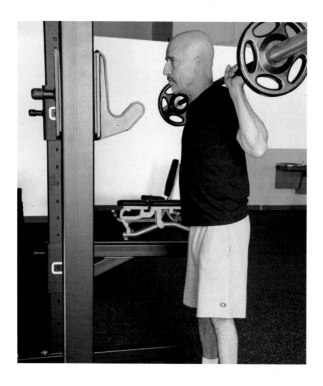

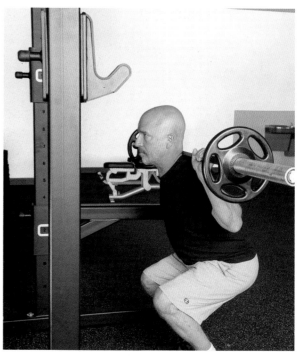

Leg Press

3 SETS 1 each of 12 reps, 10 reps, and 8 reps

⚫━⚫ **Equipment needed:** leg press machine

This exercise works your quadriceps, hamstrings, and gluteal muscles while you sit in a leg press machine and press the weight upward at a 45-degree angle.

1 Sit in the leg press machine with your back firmly against the pad and your feet on the plate about shoulder width apart. Release the safety handles to lower the weight.

2 With controlled movement, lower the weight by bending at the knees and hips, bringing your thighs toward your chest, and keeping your knees aligned with your toes.

3 To complete the repetition, contract your quadriceps muscles and press the weight back to the starting position.

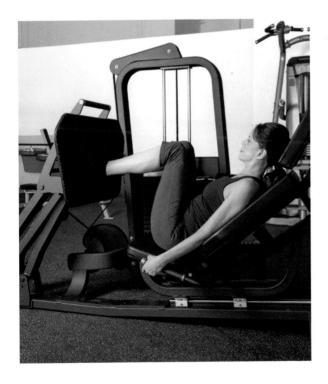
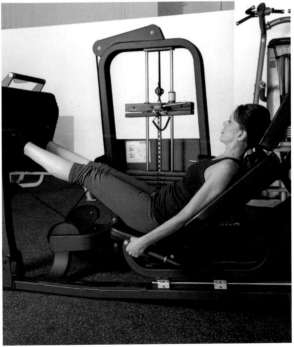

Walking Lunge

3 SETS ▶ 10 reps each

 Equipment needed: fixed-weight barbell or bar (with or without weight plates), or dumbbells

This exercise works your quadriceps, hamstrings, and gluteal muscles while you walk in long lunging steps with a barbell (or bar) balanced across your upper back and shoulders or dumbbells held at the sides of your body.

1 With a barbell or bar across your upper back, or dumbbells at your side, take a long step forward and lower your hips toward the floor until the knee of the trailing leg makes slight contact with the floor. The knee of the lead leg should be directly above the ankle (not the toes) to avoid stress on the knee.

2 Step forward with the trailing leg to a standing position.

3 Pause for balance before stepping forward with the same leg in a walking motion for the next repetition.

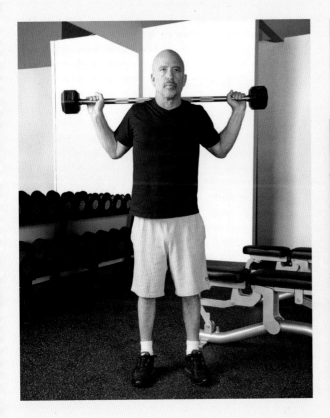 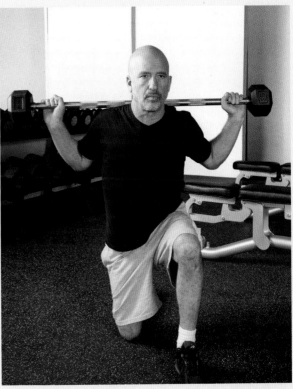

Seated Leg Curl

3 SETS ▶ 10 to 12 reps each

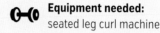 **Equipment needed:**
seated leg curl machine

This exercise works your hamstring muscles while you sit in a leg curl machine with your legs extended in front of your body and curl the weight under the seat.

1 Sit in the machine with your back pressed firmly against the pad. Your feet will be straight in front with the pad behind your ankles. The knee joint should be in alignment with the machine's pivot point.

2 To perform the repetition, contract your hamstring muscles and lower the weight, with controlled movement, to a position under the seat.

3 With controlled movement, return the weight to the starting position to complete the repetition.

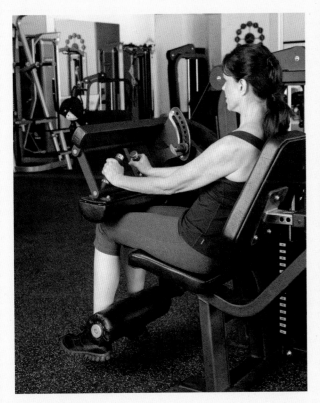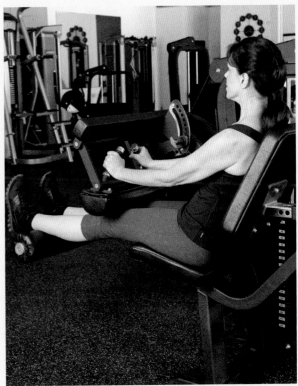

Stiff Leg Dead Lift

3 SETS 10 to 12 reps each

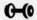 **Equipment needed:** fixed-weight barbell or bar (with or without weight plates)

This exercise works your hamstring and gluteal muscles while holding a barbell or bar in front of your body and pushing your hips backward to lower it toward the floor while avoiding bending at your knees.

1 Start from an upright position with your feet 6 to 8 in (15 to 20 cm) apart and your lower back tucked in to avoid injury. Your knees should be unlocked and your legs just slightly bent in a stiff but not "straight" position.

2 Push your hips backward and bring your shoulders down. Keep your shoulders pulled back and the back flat while hanging the barbell or bar at arm's length and close to your body.

3 To complete the repetition, contract your upper leg muscles (gluteals and hamstrings) and return to an upright position.

 ## To Perform an Inner Thigh Adduction in a Wheelchair

1 Insert your left foot into the resistance band's handle, making sure it's secure. Place the band under the right wheel for resistance.

2 Sit tall in your wheelchair without leaning into the back.

3 Extend your left leg, slowly bring it toward the center of the body, and then return it to the starting position while keeping your toes pointed toward the ceiling.

4 Repeat the exercise, this time with the resistance band handle on your right foot and the band under the left wheel.

 ## To Perform an Outer Thigh Abduction in a Wheelchair

1 Place the band's handle on your left foot, making sure it's secure. Place the band under the right wheel for resistance.

2 Sit tall in your wheelchair without leaning into the back of the wheelchair.

3 Extend your left leg, slowly bring it outward, and then return it to the starting position while keeping your toes pointed toward the ceiling.

4 Repeat the exercise, this time with the resistance band handle on your right foot and the band under the left wheel.

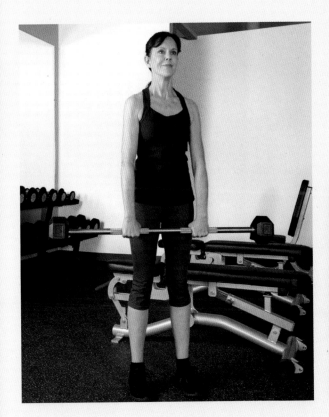 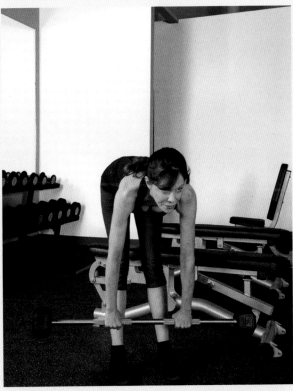

Standing Calf Raise

4 SETS   15 to 25 reps each

 Equipment needed: Smith machine and bar (with or without weight plates)

This exercise works your calf muscles, with an emphasis on the gastrocnemius muscle, while you support a weight on your shoulders in an upright position and extend your ankles to stand up on your toes.

1 Stand in the Smith machine with the weight supported on your shoulders and the balls of your feet on a platform. (You can use two weight plates as the platform.)

2 Keeping your knees in an unlocked position, press the weight up by rising up onto your toes until your calf muscles are fully contracted.

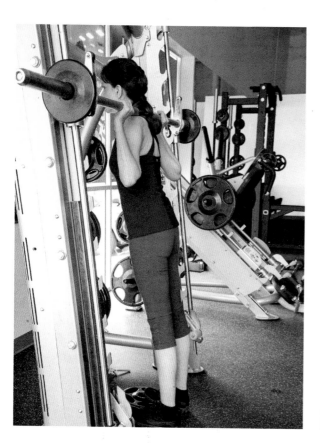
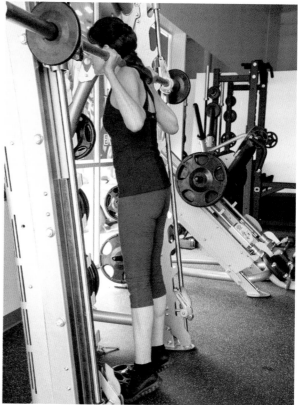

Leg Press Calf Raise

3 SETS — 15 to 25 reps each

Equipment needed:
leg press machine

This exercise works the calf muscles, with an emphasis on the gastrocnemius muscle, while supporting the sled of a leg press machine on the balls of your feet and extending your ankles.

1 Sit in the leg press machine and place the balls of your feet on the platform.

2 Keeping your knees in an unlocked position, press the weight by pushing up on your toes until your calf muscles are fully contracted.

3 To complete the repetition, lower your weight to a point where your heels are below your toes to a fully stretched position of your calf muscles.

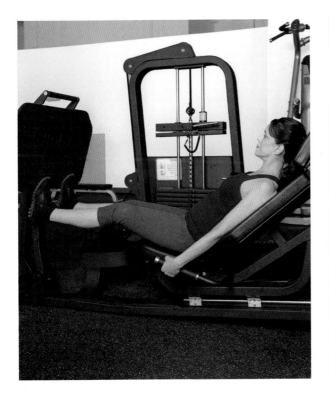
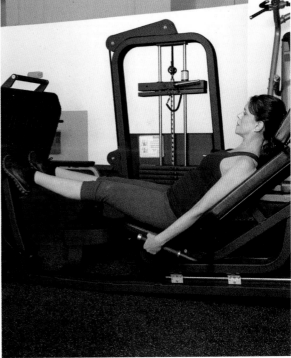

Seated Calf Raise

3 SETS ▸ 15 to 25 reps each

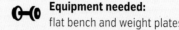 **Equipment needed:**
flat bench and weight plates

This exercise works the calf muscles, with an emphasis on the soleus muscle, while extending the ankles to raise the weight in a seated position with knees bent to 90 degrees.

1 Sit on the edge of the bench with a suitable weight plate placed across your thighs near your knees, and the balls of your feet on the edge of two weight plates on the floor.

2 Press the weight up by "standing up" on your toes until your calf muscles are fully contracted.

3 To complete the repetition, lower the weight to a point where your heels are back on the floor and below your toes to a fully stretched position of the calf muscles.

 To Perform a Calf Raise in a Wheelchair

1 Place the middle of the resistance band around your left foot, holding the handles in both hands securely with your elbows at your sides.

2 Extend your leg.

3 Point the toes forward and then slowly return to the starting position. Keep the band tight and concentrate on flexing and pointing the toes.

4 Repeat on the opposite side.

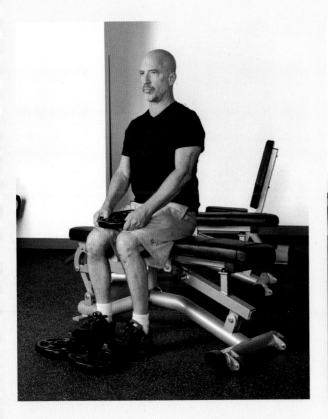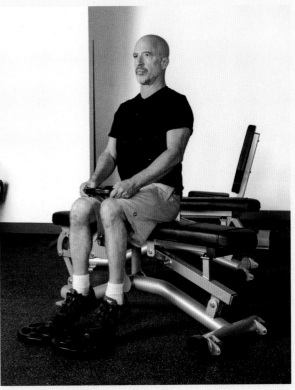

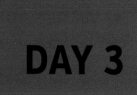

DAY 3

BACK, BICEPS, AND ABS

In Day 3 of this phase, we will be focusing on the back, biceps, and abdominal muscles. Both pulldown and rowing motions encourage complete development of the back muscles. The biceps are worked on the same day as the back muscles because they are the secondary muscles used in any back movement. The abdominal exercises will be the same as the ones performed in Phase 1, Day 1 of the program (pages 88 to 93).

Pull-Ups or Assisted Pull-Ups

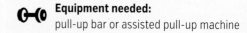

2 SETS   8 to 10 reps each   **Equipment needed:** pull-up bar or assisted pull-up machine

Pull-ups are one of the best exercises to work the back muscles, with an emphasis on the lats. They also work the shoulder and biceps muscles while starting from a full hang position and pulling the body upward.

The assisted pull-up is performed while kneeling on an assisted pull-up machine in a full hang position and pulling the body upward, allowing the machine to assist with a portion of the body weight.

1 Grasp a pull-up bar with a wide grip and hang at a full arm's length.

2 To perform the repetition, pull your body weight up to a position where your chin is above the bar, keeping your back arched and your chest up.

3 With controlled movement, lower your body to the starting position at a fully extended position to complete the repetition.

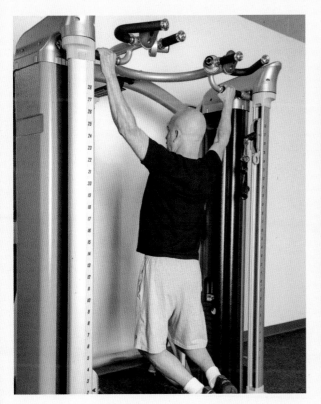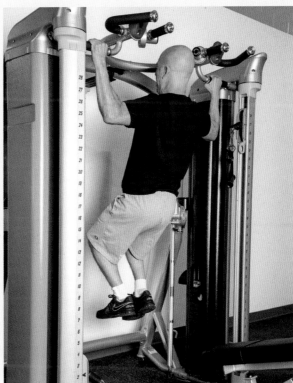

Seated Cable Row

3 SETS 1 each of 12 reps, 10 reps, and 8 reps

 Equipment needed: cable row machine with V-handle attachment

This exercise works the back muscles, with an emphasis on the lower portion of the lat muscles and rhomboids, as well as the biceps, while seated in a cable row machine and pulling the weight in a rowing motion toward the body.

1 Sit on the bench with your feet pressed firmly against the supports and your knees slightly bent. Keep your lower back tucked in and grasp the handle in front of your body.

2 To perform the repetition, pull the weight toward your midsection while simultaneously pushing your chest forward and pulling your shoulders back.

3 Return to a fully stretched position.

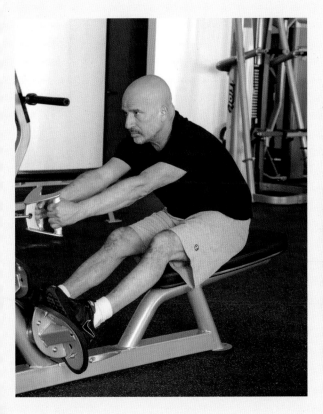 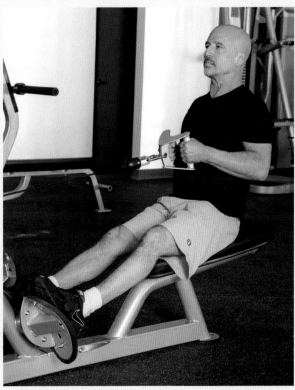

Wide-Grip Lat Pulldown

3 SETS 1 each of 12 reps, 10 reps, and 8 reps

 Equipment needed: lat pulldown machine and wide-grip lat bar attachment

This exercise works the back muscles, with an emphasis on the lats, as well as the shoulders and biceps, while pulling a weight from overhead toward the upper chest.

1 Sit in the machine with the pad across your thighs and a wider-than-shoulder-width grip on the bar.

2 To perform the repetition, lean back slightly and pull the bar toward your upper chest while bringing your elbows back 45 degrees.

3 Push your chest up toward the bar and pull your shoulders back as you pull the weight down.

4 With controlled movement, return the weight to a fully extended position to complete the repetition.

 ## To Perform a Lower Back Extension in a Wheelchair

1 Place the resistance band under the wheels and grasp each handle.

2 Bend forward from your waist until your back is parallel to the floor. Keep your elbows bent and tucked into the sides of your waist.

3 Keeping your spine as straight as possible, bend backward from your waist to sit back up and then slowly lower back down to the starting position.

4 Keep your abs and your spine lengthened. Move your feet closer to the handles to make the exercise harder, and closer to the center of the band to make it easier. *Remember, to avoid back injury you must do these exercises slowly and without jerking your back.*

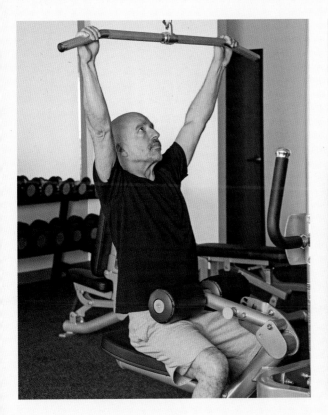 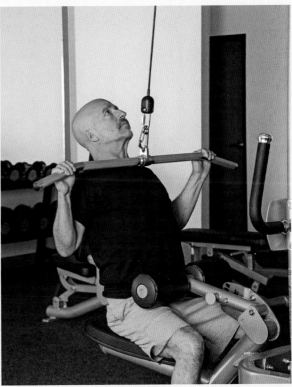

Barbell Row

3 SETS | 10 to 12 reps each

 Equipment needed: fixed-weight barbell or bar (with or without weight plates)

This exercise works the mid-back muscles, with an emphasis on the rhomboids and lats, as well as the shoulders and biceps, while holding a barbell or bar in front of the body in a slightly bent-over position and pulling it toward the body.

1 Stand with your feet at shoulder width and your knees slightly bent.

2 Start with the bar hanging at arm's length, with a shoulder-width grip.

3 Bend forward at the waist until your upper body is almost parallel to the floor, keeping your lower back tucked in to avoid injury.

4 To perform the repetition, push your chest toward the floor and pull your shoulders back as you pull the bar to your lower rib area and then return the bar, with controlled movement, to a full arm's length.

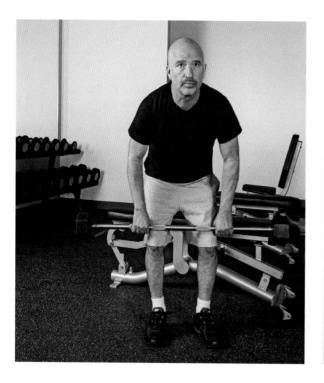

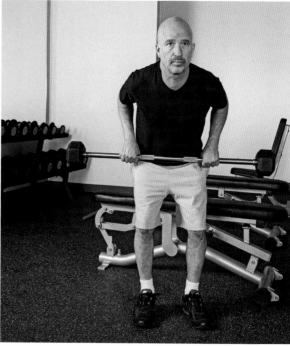

Straight-Arm Lat Pulldown

2 SETS 10 to 12 reps each

Equipment needed: cable machine with pulley in the high position and wide-grip lat bar attachment

This exercise works the back muscles, with an emphasis on the lats, trapezius, and shoulders, while lowering a weight in an arcing motion from an extended position toward the thighs.

1 Stand facing the high cable machine with your feet together, knees slightly bent, and lower back tucked in to prevent injury. Lean slightly forward and grip the bar with a wider-than-shoulder-width grip and your elbows slightly bent.

2 To perform the repetition, bring the weight down in an arcing motion toward your thighs, keeping your elbows from bending and moving only at your shoulder.

3 At the bottom of the movement, raise your chest and pull your shoulders back. Maintain a slightly forward angle of your upper body and avoid standing upright.

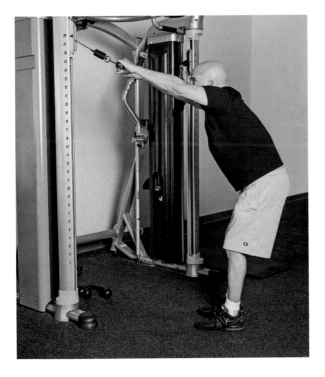
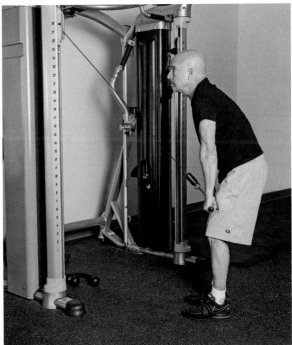

Barbell Curl

3 SETS — 1 each of 12 reps, 10 reps, and 8 reps

 Equipment needed: mixed-weight barbell or bar (with or without weight plates)

This exercise works the biceps muscles while holding a barbell or bar in front of the body with arms hanging downward and curling the weight up toward the shoulders.

1 Stand with your feet approximately shoulder width apart, knees slightly bent, and core tight. Grasp the bar with a shoulder-width grip, palms facing away from your body.

2 To perform the repetition, contract your biceps and curl the bar up toward your shoulders.

3 At the top position, squeeze your biceps before lowering the weight to the starting position. Avoid swinging your weight to prevent lower back injuries.

 To Perform a Biceps Curl in a Wheelchair

1 Secure the resistance band by looping it under the wheelchair wheels.

2 With arms down at your sides, grab the resistance band handles.

3 Keeping your elbows at your sides and palms facing outward, slowly raise your hands toward your shoulders and then slowly return them to the starting position. Keep your wrists in line with your forearms, not bent.

4 With a slight variation of turning your palms in toward your legs, the biceps curl now becomes a seated hammer curl. This movement is used primarily to target the biceps, and because your wrists remain perpendicular to the ground rather than parallel, your forearms also get a workout.

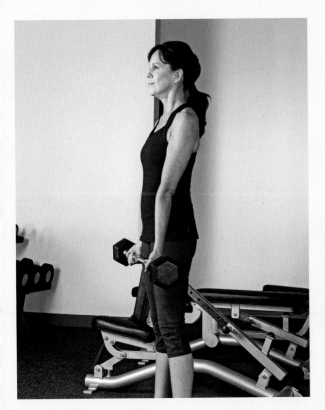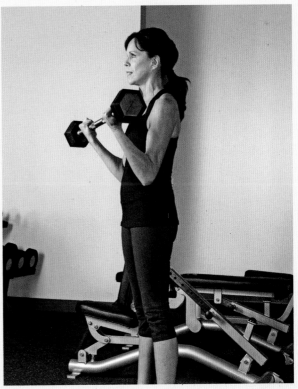

Incline Dumbbell Curl

3 SETS　10 to 12 reps each

 Equipment needed:
incline or adjustable bench and dumbbells

This exercise works the biceps muscles, with an emphasis on the long head of the muscle, while seated on an inclined bench and curling the weight from a hanging position upward toward your shoulders.

1 Sit on an adjustable bench angled back approximately 45 degrees. Begin with a dumbbell in each hand and let your arms hang at your sides with your palms facing forward.

2 Squeeze your biceps and curl the weight up toward your shoulders.

3 With controlled movement, lower the weight back to the starting position to complete the repetition.

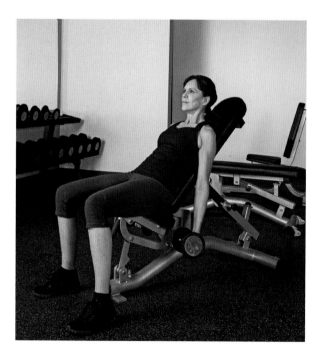 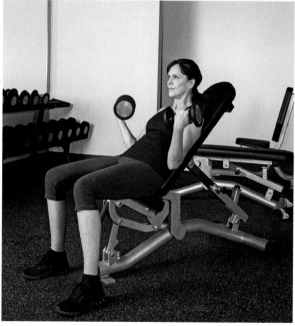

Rope Hammer Curl

3 SETS 10 to 12 reps each

Equipment needed: cable machine with pulley in the low position and rope attachment

For this exercise, you may choose to perform the rope hammer curl or preacher curl (page 120). The rope hammer curl works the biceps muscles, with an emphasis on the short head of the muscle, as well as the brachialis muscle, while curling a weight up toward the shoulders with a rope attachment connected to a low pulley.

1 Stand facing the cable machine, keeping your knees unlocked and your core muscles tight. Grasp the rope with a thumbs-up grip and your elbows slightly in front of your body.

2 To perform the repetition, squeeze your biceps and curl the weight up toward your shoulders while keeping the thumbs-up hand position and elbows in front of your body.

3 With controlled movement, lower the weight to the starting position to complete the repetition. Avoid swinging the weight to prevent lower back injuries.

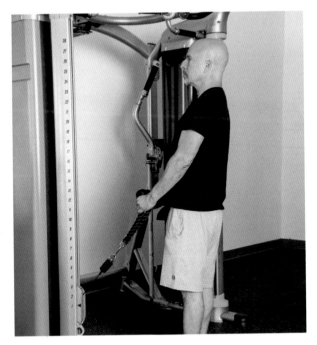 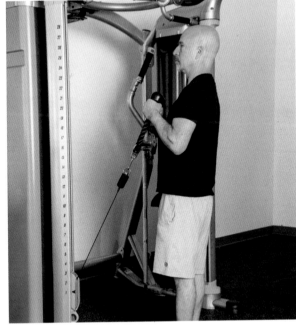

Preacher Curl

3 SETS   10 to 12 reps each

Equipment needed: preacher curl machine or preacher curl bench with fixed-weight barbell or E-Z curl bar

Instead of the rope hammer curl, you may choose to perform the preacher curl. This exercise works your biceps, with an emphasis on the short head of the muscle, as you curl a weight toward your shoulders with your elbows supported in front of your body on a preacher bench.

1 Sit in the machine with your arms over the pad and your elbows in line with your shoulders. Grasp the bar or handles with a palms-up grip.

2 To perform the repetition, squeeze your biceps as you curl the weight up toward your shoulders while keeping your elbows in contact with the pad.

3 With controlled movement, lower the weight back to the starting position to complete the repetition. Avoid overextending your elbows to prevent injury.

Repeat the ab routine on Phase 1, Day 1 (pages 90 to 93): (1) knee tuck, hip thrust, or leg raise; (2) crunch; (3) medicine ball Russian twist

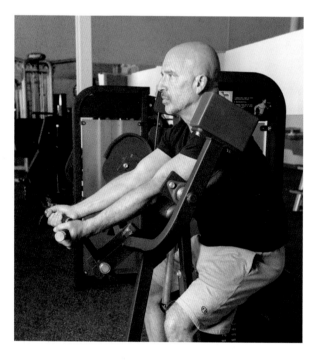
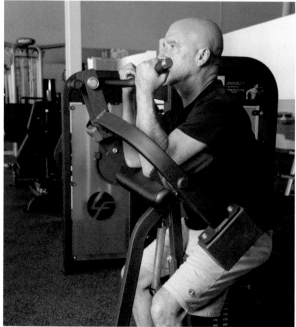

CHAPTER 6

Phase 2
Jump-Start Your Metabolism

Phase 2 is where you will begin to see major progress. You've laid the groundwork in Phase 1, and now it's time to kick things into high gear. If you've made it this far, your confidence should be riding high, and it's time for even bigger results! There are a few elements of this phase to know before you begin.

Phase 2 introduces metabolism jump-start options. These are multi-joint movements used as active rest between sets to add a cardio component to the workout, increase endurance, and help burn additional calories. These are body weight movements. With the exception of jumping rope (if you choose this option), no additional equipment is necessary.

Some exercises in this phase are also in Phase 1, while others are new. The program is broken down further to alternate different workouts on a weekly basis, providing a change in routine and a variety of exercises to help keep the body from adapting to the workout. As with Phase 1, this workout can be performed for more than three days per week, but due to the higher intensity of the workouts, three days may be sufficient for many people.

METABOLISM JUMP-START

Metabolism jump-starts replace your rest periods between sets. The point is to keep moving for an entire minute before beginning the next set. For people just beginning this phase, you might start with 20 to 30 seconds and rest the remainder of the minute before starting the next set, until you develop the cardiovascular conditioning to perform the movement for the entire minute. Choose one exercise from the lists on pages 122 and 123, and keep each minute as intense as possible. As you progress, your intensity level will increase.

Air Squat (Body Weight Squat)

An air squat is simply a squat performed using your own body weight.

- Perform a regular squat without any additional weight.
- At the bottom of the squat, make sure your hips are below your knees to allow for maximum engagement of your glutes and hamstring muscles.

Jump Squat (Plyometric Squat)

A jump squat is quite similar to an air squat, but with an explosive jump.

- Begin by performing a regular squat without any additional weight.
- Instead of simply rising out of the squat back to a standing position, rise into a jump feet several inches (10 to 15 cm) off the floor.
- Upon landing from the jump, make a smooth descent into the next squat.

Step-Ups

Keeping minimal weight on the stepping foot, simply touch your foot lightly on the bench to keep maximum tension on your muscles.

- Standing in front of a step or a bench, place one foot on the step and keep it there until all repetitions on that side are complete.
- With the other foot, step up onto the bench, shifting your weight onto the step.
- Step back down with the stepping foot to complete the repetition.
- When the repetitions are complete, repeat by stepping with the other foot.

Running in Place

It's as simple as it sounds!

- Run in place, raising your knees up high, to raise your heart rate.

Alternating Body Weight Lunges

- From a normal standing position, with your hands on your hips, take a long step forward into a lunge position. At the full lunge position, your front leg should be bent to a 90-degree angle with your knee directly over your ankle. Your back knee should bend until it lightly touches the floor. Your upper body should remain upright and your hips should drop straight down.

- To return to the starting position, push back off your front foot and return your body to a normal standing position. Repeat the movement on your other side to complete the repetition.

Mountain Climber

- Start in a push-up or plank position with both palms on the floor and arms extended underneath your shoulders, legs extended straight back with the balls of your feet resting on the floor.

- To perform the repetition, bring one knee toward your chest.

- Continue by driving that foot back to the starting position while simultaneously bringing the opposite knee toward your chest in a running motion.

Jump Rope

Technique can vary according to an individual's skill level. This can include single jumps, double jumps, or running in place, for example.

- With the correct length of jump rope (avoid dragging too much on the ground, and avoid tripping on it or hitting your head), jump 30 seconds to 1 minute between sets to keep the heart rate elevated.

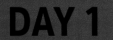

DAY 1

CHEST, TRICEPS, AND ABS

On Day 1 of Phase 2, we work the chest, triceps, and abdominal muscles. Triceps are grouped with the chest because they are the secondary muscle used in all chest movements. Even though Phase 1 has prepared you for this phase, we still recommend you use a spotter, when possible. People who experience symptoms of fatigue or overheating should be particularly careful when training in this phase.

Chest Press

4 SETS

8 to 12 reps each

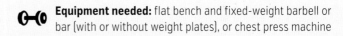 **Equipment needed:** flat bench and fixed-weight barbell or bar (with or without weight plates), or chest press machine

This exercise can be performed on a flat bench or using a chest press machine. The flat bench chest press works the chest muscles, as well as the shoulders and triceps, while lifting a bar over the chest. The machine chest press works the chest muscles, with an emphasis on the middle chest, as well as the shoulders and triceps, while pressing the machine's handles forward in front of the body in an upright, seated position.

1 Lying flat on the bench, start with the barbell or bar extended over your chest.

2 To perform the repetition, with controlled movement, lower the weight to a point where the weight is in line with the center of your chest.

3 Pause, and then flex your chest muscles to press the weight back to a fully extended position.

4 Squeeze your chest muscles before lowering the weight for the next repetition.

5 To perform this on a chest press machine, see Phase 1, machine chest press (page 72), for exercise description and required equipment.

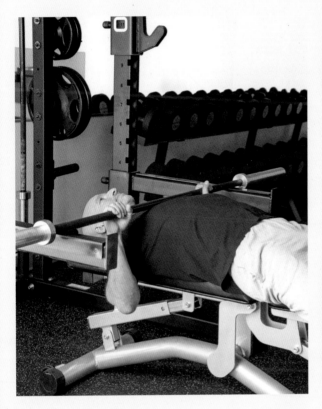
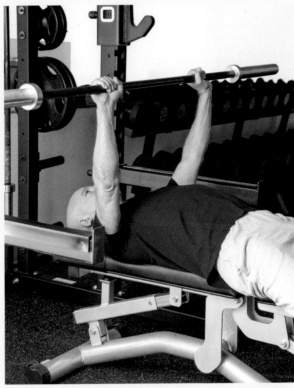

Incline Bench Press with Dumbbells

3 SETS ➤ 8 to 12 reps each

 Equipment needed: Smith machine with bar or incline bench with dumbbells

This exercise works the chest muscles, with an emphasis on the upper chest, as well as the shoulders and triceps, while either lifting a bar (with or without weight plates), supported by the Smith machine, or dumbbells, over the chest. You have a choice of equipment and can alternate these, as you desire. See page 71 for photos of the Smith machine incline bench press with a bar.

1 If you are using an adjustable bench, set the incline at approximately 30 degrees, which is the optimal angle to work the upper chest.

2 Grip the bar or dumbbells with a slightly wider-than-shoulder-width grip. The starting position should be across the upper chest.

3 Squeeze the muscles of your chest as you press the weight over your chest. If using dumbbells, bring the dumbbells together over your chest as you press upward.

4 With controlled movement, return the weight to the starting position to complete the repetition. Avoid letting the weight just fall back to the starting position or bounce off your chest to begin the next rep because this can cause injury.

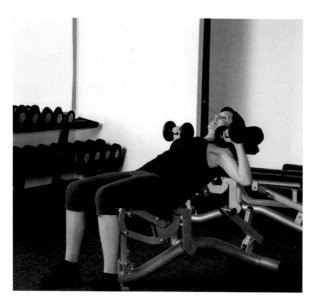
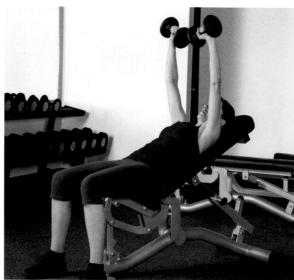

Pec Deck Fly

3 SETS   8 to 12 reps each

Equipment needed: pec deck machine

This exercise works the chest muscles, with an emphasis on the outer chest during the stretch position and the inner chest during the contracted position, as well as the shoulders, while starting in a wide, arms outstretched position and moving to a contracted position in front of the body.

1 Sit in the pec deck machine. Starting with your arms outstretched and elbows slightly bent, contract your chest muscles as you bring the weight forward in an arcing motion until your hands come together in front of your chest.

2 Squeeze your chest muscles and then return the handles to the starting position in a reverse arcing motion. Keep a slight bend in your elbows to avoid overextending your shoulder.

3 Also, keep the bend in your elbows at a minimum to avoid engaging your biceps in the movement.

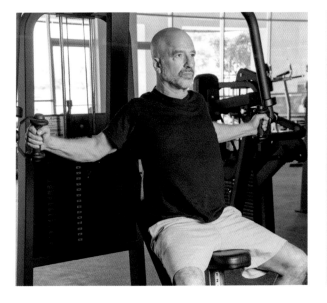
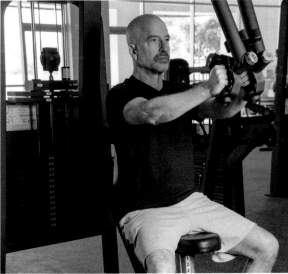

Bench Dip

4 SETS ▸ 8 to 12 reps each

Equipment needed:
flat bench

Perform the bench dip while seated and fully extend your arms to lift yourself off the bench. Working your triceps, lower your body off the side of the bench and then return to a fully extended arm position to raise your body back up.

1 Sit on the bench with your feet out in front of you resting on your heels with only a slight bend in your knees. Place your hands on the bench, palms down and fingers facing forward toward your feet.

2 Move your hips forward, off the bench, so your body weight is supported on your hands. Keep your lower back tucked in and chest up for good posture.

3 With controlled movement, lower your body weight until your upper arms are bent 90 degrees.

4 Keep your back close to the bench to avoid unnecessary stress on the shoulder joint and press upward, back to the original starting position, while contracting your triceps muscles.

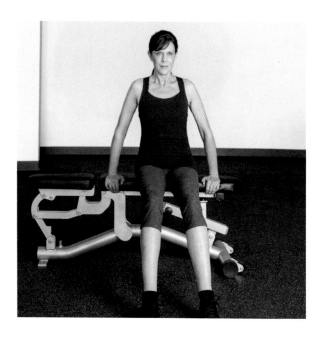
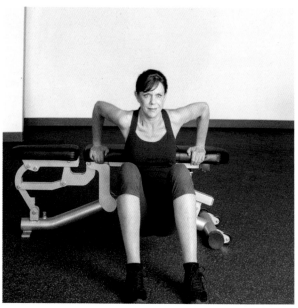

Close-Grip Bench Press

4 SETS

8 to 12 reps each

Equipment needed: flat bench, Smith machine with bar (with or without weight plates), or fixed-weight barbell

This exercise works the triceps muscles, as well as the chest and shoulders, while pressing a bar (supported by a Smith machine) over the chest with a closer than normal grip on the bar.

1 Lie on a flat bench under the Smith machine. Grip the bar with your hands approximately 10 to 12 in (25 to 30 cm) apart.

2 Keep your elbows close to your ribs as the weight is lowered and then press straight up without letting your elbows flare out, keeping the tension on your triceps.

3 With controlled movement, lower the weight to the starting position.

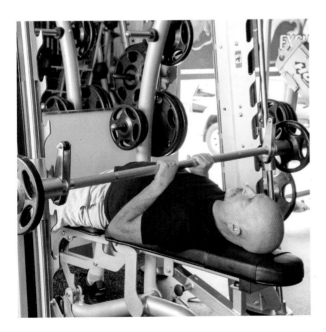
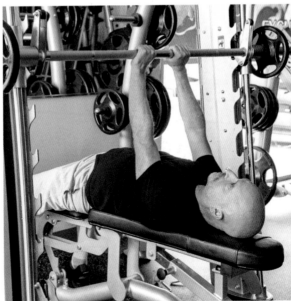

Cable Crunch

3 SETS   12 to 15 reps each

 Equipment needed: cable machine with pulley in the high position, rope attachment

You may choose to perform the cable crunch or the weighted crunch, opposite. The cable crunch works the abdominal muscles with a crunching motion while holding a weight attached to a high pulley.

1 Kneel in front of a high cable machine. Using a rope attachment, set the desired weight and hold both ends of the rope at the sides of your head.

2 Keeping this position with your elbows near your ribs, roll your shoulders toward your knees in a crunching motion while contracting your abdominal muscles to complete the repetition. Keep your lower back tucked in and return your shoulders to the starting position.

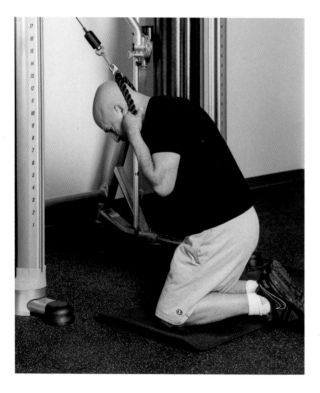

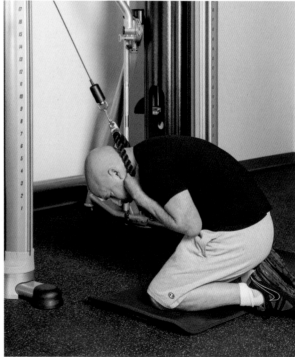

Weighted Crunch

3 SETS

12 to 15 reps each

Equipment needed:
weight plate, dumbbell, or kettlebell

Instead of the cable crunch, opposite, you may perform the weighted crunch, which works the abdominal muscles while holding on to a weight plate, dumbbell, or kettlebell for added resistance. The weighted crunch is performed in the same manner as a regular crunch (page 92), except your arms are extended above your chest to hold a weight at full arm's length.

1 Lie flat on the floor with your knees bent and feet flat on the floor. With the weight in hand, extend your arms above your chest to hold the weight at full arm's length.

2 To perform the repetition, press your lower back into the floor and raise your shoulders, pushing the weight toward the ceiling, and then return to the starting position.

Leg Raise to Hip Thrust

3 SETS 12 to 15 reps each

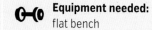 **Equipment needed:**
flat bench

You may choose to perform the leg raise to hip thrust or the reverse crunch, opposite. The leg raise to hip thrust works the lower portion of the abdominal muscles while raising the legs 90 degrees and then raising the hips to push the feet toward the ceiling.

1 Lie on the bench and grasp the sides of it near your head.

2 Extend your legs and raise them 90 degrees while keeping your knees locked.

3 At 90 degrees, push your feet toward the ceiling and raise your hips several inches (10 to 15 cm) off the bench to engage your lower ab muscles.

4 Lower your hips to the bench while keeping your legs straight up toward the ceiling to complete the repetition.

5 Keep your knees locked and lower your legs from a 90-degree position back to fully extended and parallel with the bench.

Reverse Crunch

3 SETS 12 to 15 reps each

Equipment needed:
flat bench

Instead of the leg raise to hip thrust, opposite, you may choose to perform the reverse crunch, which works the lower portion of the abdominal muscles while bringing the knees toward the chest to roll the hips upward.

1 Lie on the bench and grasp the sides of it near your head.

2 With your legs fully extended, draw your knees toward your chest and allow your hips to roll up off the bench to engage your lower abdominal muscles.

3 Push your feet forward to a fully extended leg position to complete the repetition.

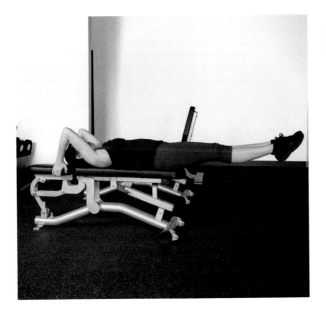

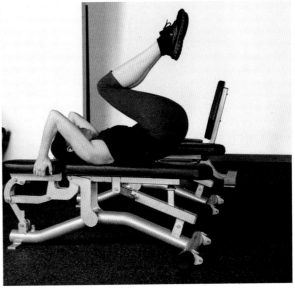

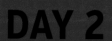

DAY 2

SHOULDERS, LEGS, AND CALVES

On Day 2 of Phase 2, we will work the shoulder, leg, and calf muscles. As always, the movement with correct form is more important than the amount of weight being used. Focusing on good form and technique and allowing the weight to progress slowly keeps the risk of injury at a minimum. We recommend the use of a spotter whenever possible. If you experience fatigue or neuropathy in your hands, be especially careful because you will work some of your larger muscles and press weights overhead, possibly leading you to experience fatigue much quicker.

Barbell Shoulder Press

4 SETS ▸ 8 to 12 reps each

 Equipment needed: fixed-weight barbell or bar (with or without weight plates)

This exercise works the shoulder muscles while pressing a barbell or bar from a racked position (a position in front of the body at shoulder level) to a fully locked out overhead position.

1 Start from a seated or standing position with a slightly wider than shoulder-width grip on a barbell or bar.

2 With the barbell or bar in front of your body at approximately the level of your collarbones, press the weight to a fully extended overhead position.

3 With controlled movement, lower the weight to the starting position to complete the repetition.

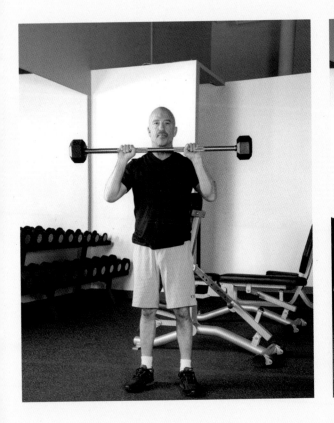 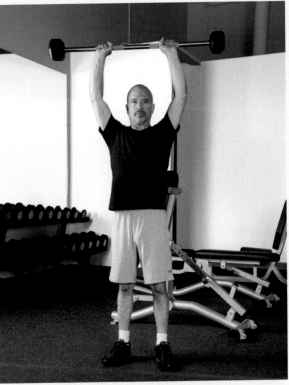

Alternating Dumbbell Shoulder Press

3 SETS 8 to 12 reps each

Equipment needed: dumbbells

You may choose to perform this exercise or the machine shoulder press, opposite. The alternating dumbbell shoulder press exercise works the shoulder muscles while pressing a dumbbell overhead in an alternating fashion—first one side and then the other.

1 With a dumbbell in each hand at approximately the level of your collarbones, press one weight overhead to a position where your arm is fully extended.

2 With controlled movement, slowly lower the weight to the starting position to complete the repetition.

3 Repeat with your other arm.

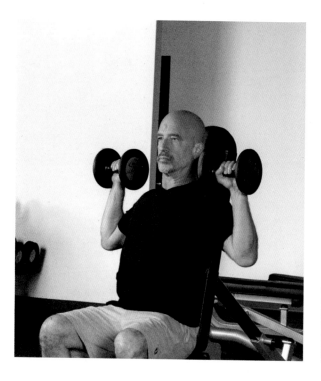
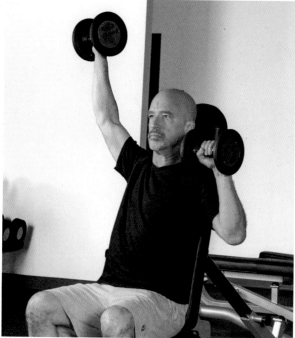

Machine Shoulder Press

3 SETS

8 to 12 reps each

⚫━⚫ **Equipment needed:** shoulder press machine (or similar arm press machine)

Instead of the alternating dumbbell shoulder press, opposite, you may perform a machine shoulder press. If you have access to a shoulder press machine with which each side can be pressed independently, then the movement will be performed in an alternating fashion, the same way as the alternating dumbbell shoulder press.

1 Using a hammer strength machine, or a similar machine that allows each arm to press independently, start with the weight at approximately the level of your collarbones and press the weight to a fully extended overhead position.

2 With controlled movement, lower the weight to the starting position to complete the repetition. The independent motion of this machine will help correct any imbalances in strength from one side to the other.

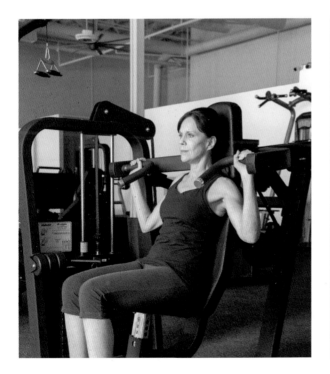

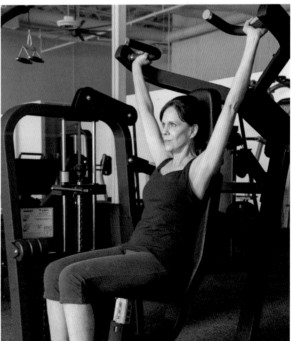

Smith Machine Upright Row

3 SETS — 8 to 12 reps each **Equipment needed:** Smith machine and bar (with or without weight plates)

You may choose to perform the Smith machine upright row or cable upright row, opposite. The Smith machine upright row works the shoulder muscles, with an emphasis on the anterior head of the muscle, as well as the upper back muscles, while raising a bar supported by the Smith machine from an arms hanging in front of the body position to underneath the chin.

1 Standing in front of a Smith machine, take a grip on the bar with your hands approximately 10 to 12 in (25 to 30 cm) apart.

2 With your knees in an unlocked position and your core muscles tight, raise the weight to a position under your chin while raising your elbows as high as possible.

3 With controlled movement, lower the weight to the starting position to complete the repetition.

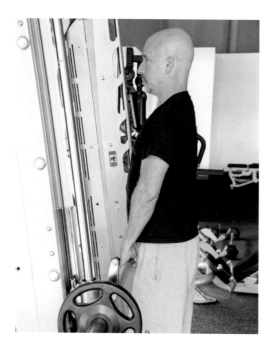

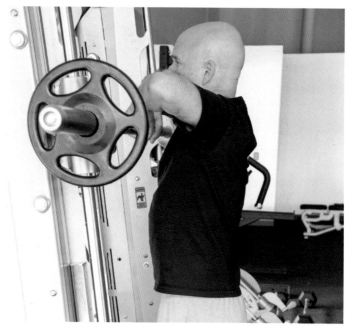

Cable Upright Row

 3 SETS   8 to 12 reps each

 Equipment needed: cable machine with pulley in the low position, with rope attachment or straight bar attachment

Instead of the Smith machine upright row, opposite, you may choose to perform the cable upright row. The cable upright row works the shoulder muscles, with an emphasis on the anterior head of the muscle, as well as the upper back muscles, in the same manner as the Smith machine upright row, but while using a rope or bar attachment connected to a low pulley.

1 This movement is performed in the same manner as the Smith machine upright row, opposite, with the only difference being that you use a rope attachment on a low pulley cable machine.

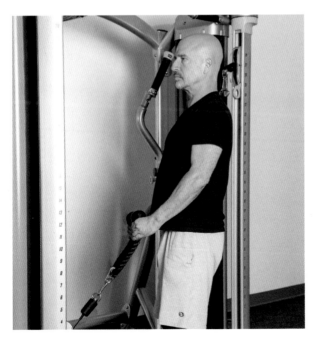
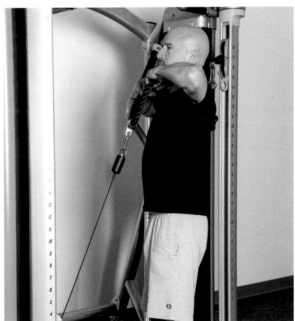

Squat

4 SETS | 8 to 12 reps each

Equipment needed: squat rack and bar (with or without weight plates)

This exercise works the quadriceps, hamstrings, and gluteal muscles while standing with a weight balanced across the upper back and shoulders and squatting to a position where the hips are below the knees.

1 Start with the bar across your upper back and your feet shoulder width apart or slightly wider.

2 Keep your lower back tucked in and your chest up as you bend at your knees and hips to a full squat position, where your hips are slightly below the knee joint. Always align the knees with the toes to avoid injury.

3 Avoid leaning forward as you return to a standing position to complete the repetition.

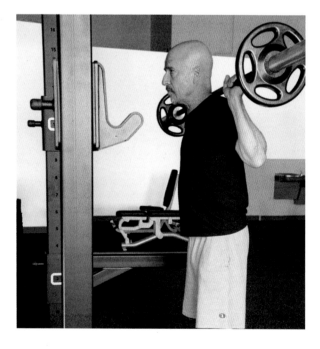

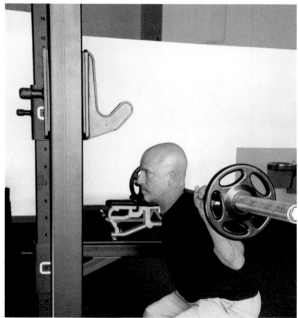

Dead Lift

3 SETS

8 to 12 reps each

 Equipment needed: fixed-weight barbell or bar (with or without weight plates)

This exercise works all the major leg muscles, including the quadriceps, hamstrings, and gluteal muscles, as well as the core muscles and back muscles, while lifting a barbell or bar off the floor to a fully upright position.

1 Starting with a barbell or bar on the floor, grasp the bar with an over/under grip (one hand with the palm facing toward the body and the other hand with palm facing away from the body), slightly wider than hip width apart.

2 With your hips low and your lower back tucked in, chest up as in a squat position, lift the weight off the floor to a standing upright position while keeping the weight as close to your body as possible.

3 With controlled movement, lower your hips, as in a squat motion, until the weight is returned to the floor to complete the repetition.

Walking Lunge

3 SETS — 10 reps each

 Equipment needed: fixed-weight barbell or bar (with or without weight plates), or dumbbells

This exercise works the quadriceps, hamstrings, and gluteal muscles while walking in long lunging steps with a barbell (or bar) balanced across the upper back and shoulders or dumbbells held at the sides of the body.

1 With a barbell or bar across your upper back, or dumbbells at the side, take a long step forward and lower your hips toward the floor until the knee of the trailing leg makes slight contact with the floor. The knee of the lead leg should be directly above the ankle (not the toes) to avoid stress on the knee.

2 Step forward with the trailing leg to a standing position.

3 Pause for balance before stepping forward with the same leg in a walking motion for the next repetition.

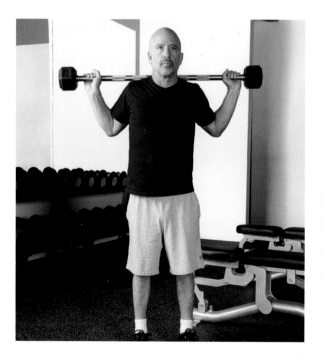

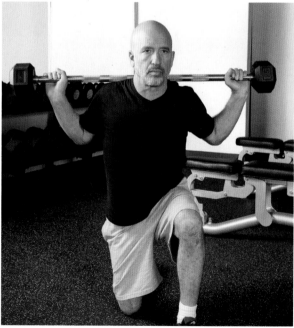

Standing Calf Raise

3 SETS

12 to 15 reps each

Equipment needed: Smith machine and bar (with or without weight plates)

This exercise works the calf muscles, with an emphasis on the gastrocnemius muscle, while supporting a weight on the shoulders in an upright position and extending the ankles to stand up on the toes.

1 Stand in the Smith machine with the weight supported on your shoulders, and the balls of your feet on a platform. (You can use two weight plates as the platform.)

2 Keeping your knees in an unlocked position, press the weight up by rising up onto your toes until your calf muscles are fully contracted.

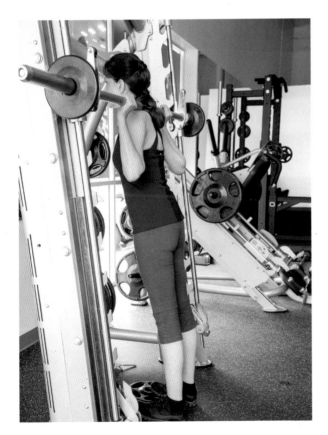
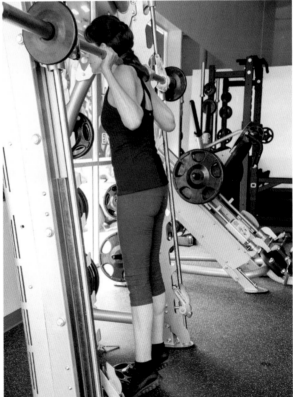

Leg Press Calf Raise

3 SETS 12 to 15 each

 Equipment needed: leg press machine

This exercise works the calf muscles, with an emphasis on the gastrocnemius muscle, while supporting the sled of a leg press machine on the balls of the feet and extending the ankles.

1 Sit in the leg press machine and place the balls of your feet on the platform.

2 Keeping your knees in an unlocked position, press the weight by pushing up on your toes until your calf muscles are fully contracted.

3 To complete the repetition, lower the weight to a point where your heels are below your toes to a fully stretched position of the calf muscles.

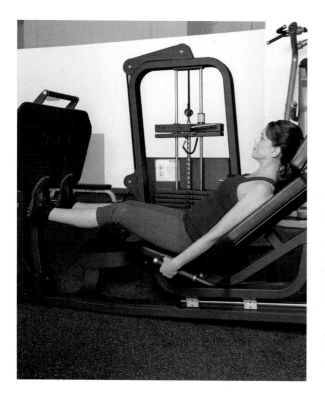 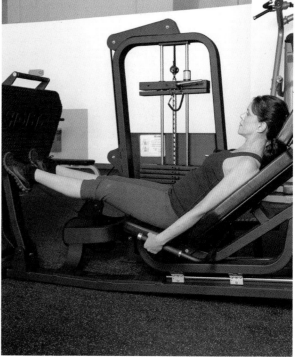

Seated Calf Raise

3 SETS 12 to 15 each

Equipment needed:
flat bench and weight plates

This exercise works the calf muscles, with an emphasis on the soleus muscle, while extending the ankles to raise the weight in a seated position with knees bent to 90 degrees.

1 Sit on the edge of the bench with a suitable weight plate placed across your thighs near your knees, and the balls of your feet on the edge of two weight plates on the floor.

2 Press the weight up by "standing up" on your toes until your calf muscles are fully contracted.

3 To complete the repetition, lower the weight to a point where your heels are back on the floor and below your toes to a fully stretched position of your calf muscles.

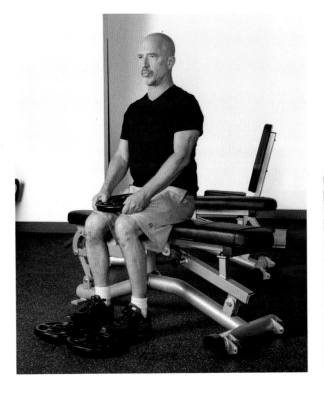
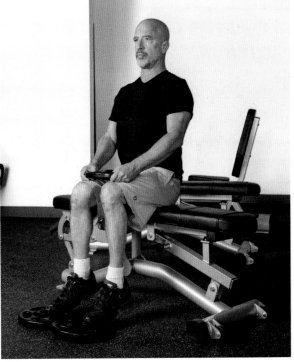

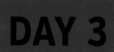
BACK, BICEPS, AND ABS

On Day 3, we are working the back, biceps, and abdominal muscles. Biceps are grouped with the back because they are the secondary muscle used in all back movements. People who experience symptoms of fatigue or neuropathy in the hands should be extremely careful when gripping a weight in an overhead position. As always, the use of a spotter is recommended for safety, when possible.

Barbell Row

4 SETS ▶ 8 to 12 reps each

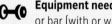 **Equipment needed:** fixed-weight barbell or bar (with or without weight plates)

This exercise works the mid-back muscles, with an emphasis on the rhomboids and lats, as well as the shoulders and biceps, while holding a barbell or bar in front of the body in a slightly bent-over position and pulling it toward the body.

1 Stand with your feet at shoulder width and your knees slightly bent.

2 Start with the bar hanging at arm's length, with a shoulder-width grip.

3 Bend forward at your waist until your upper body is almost parallel to the floor, keeping your lower back tucked in to avoid injury.

4 To perform the repetition, push your chest toward the floor and pull your shoulders back as you pull the bar to the lower rib area, and then return the bar, with controlled movement, to a full arm's length.

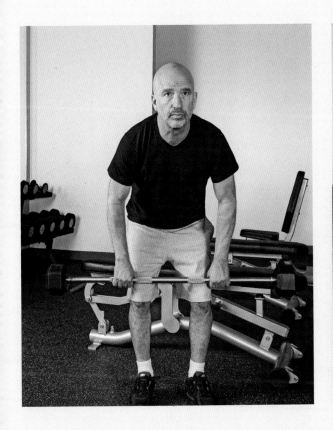 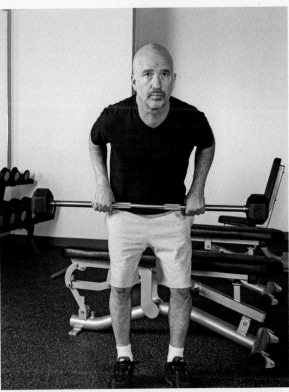

Wide-Grip Lat Pulldown

3 SETS ▶ 8 to 12 reps each

 Equipment needed: flat pulldown machine and wide-grip lat bar attachment

This exercise works the back muscles, with an emphasis on the lats, as well as the shoulders and biceps, while pulling a weight from overhead toward the upper chest.

1 Sit in the machine with the pad across your thighs and a wider-than-shoulder-width grip on the bar.

2 To perform the repetition, lean back slightly and pull the bar toward your upper chest while bringing your elbows back 45 degrees.

3 Push your chest up toward the bar and pull your shoulders back as you pull the weight down.

4 With controlled movement, return the weight to a fully extended position to complete the repetition.

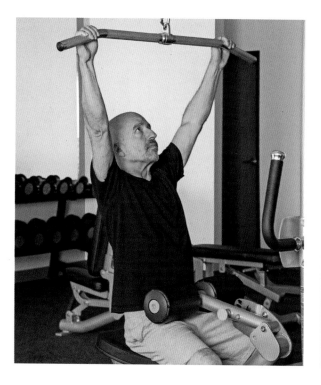
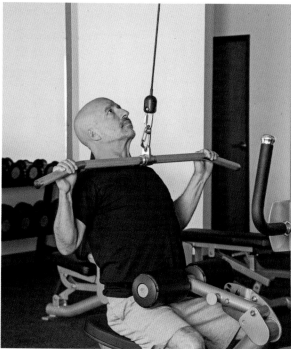

Seated Cable Row

3 SETS

8 to 12 reps each

Equipment needed:
cable row machine with V-handle attachment

This exercise works the back muscles, with an emphasis on the lower portion of the lat muscles and the rhomboids, as well as the biceps, while seated in a cable row machine and pulling the weight in a rowing motion toward the body.

1 Sit on the bench with your feet pressed firmly against the supports and your knees slightly bent. Keep your lower back tucked in and grasp the handle in front of your body.

2 To perform the repetition, pull the weight toward your midsection while simultaneously pushing your chest forward and pulling your shoulders back.

3 Return to a fully stretched position.

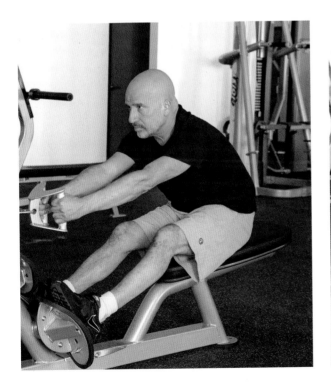
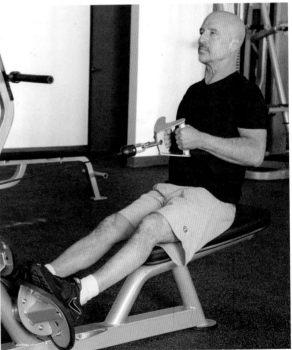

Barbell Curl

3 SETS — 8 to 12 reps each

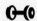 **Equipment needed:** fixed-weight barbell or bar (with or without weight plates)

This exercise works the biceps muscles while holding a barbell or bar in front of the body with arms hanging downward and curling the weight up toward the shoulders.

1 Stand with your feet approximately shoulder-width apart, knees slightly bent, and core tight. Grasp the bar with a shoulder-width grip, palms facing away from your body.

2 To perform the repetition, contract your biceps and curl the bar up toward your shoulders.

3 At the top position, squeeze your biceps before lowering the weight to the starting position. Avoid swinging the weight to prevent lower back injuries.

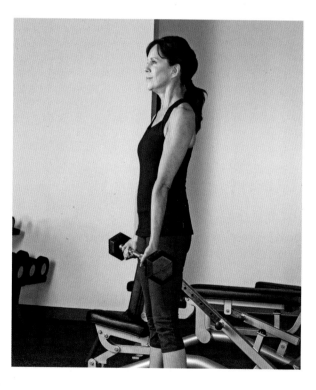

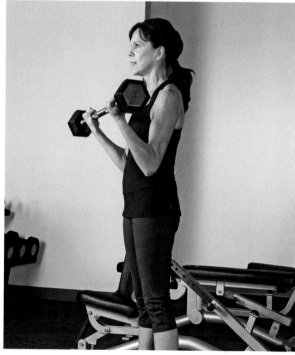

Preacher Curl with Dumbbells

3 SETS · 8 to 12 reps each

Equipment needed: preacher curl bench, dumbbells, and E-Z curl bar or preacher curl machine

The preacher curl works the biceps muscles, with an emphasis on the short head of the muscle, while curling a weight toward the shoulders with the elbows supported in front of the body on a preacher bench. The machine preacher curl allows the additional safety of a machine and eliminates the need to balance the weights.

1 Sitting in a preacher curl bench with your upper arms and elbows resting on the pad and a dumbbell in each hand, flex your biceps and curl the dumbbells toward your shoulders while maintaining your elbow's contact with the machine's pad. Curl dumbbells simultaneously or alternating.

2 Also, keep a distance of at least 1 in (2.5 cm) between the dumbbells to avoid having them make contact.

3 With controlled movement, lower the weight to the starting position. Stop short of your elbows being completely locked out to avoid unnecessary stress or hyperextension of the elbow joint and complete the repetition.

Cable Crunch

3 SETS   12 to 15 reps each

Equipment needed: cable machine with pulley in the high position, rope attachment

You may choose to perform the cable crunch or the weighted crunch, opposite. The cable crunch works the abdominal muscles with a crunching motion while holding a weight attached to a high pulley.

1 Kneel in front of a high cable machine. Using a rope attachment, set the desired weight and hold both ends of the rope at the sides of your head.

2 Keeping the rope in this position and your elbows near your ribs, roll your shoulders toward your knees in a crunching motion while contracting your abdominal muscles to complete the repetition. Keep your lower back tucked in and return your shoulders to the starting position.

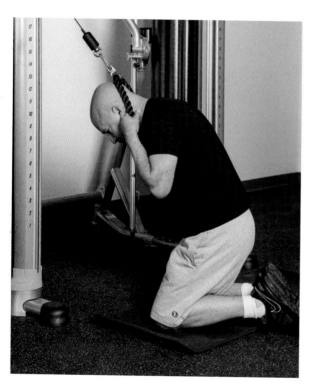
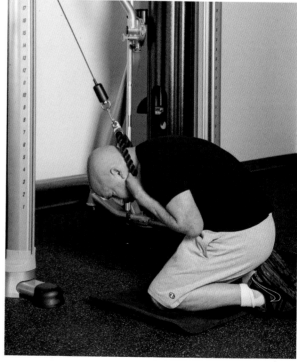

Weighted Crunch

3 SETS

12 to 15 reps each

Equipment needed:
weight plate, dumbbell, or kettlebell

Instead of the cable crunch, opposite, you may choose to perform the weighted crunch, which works the abdominal muscles while holding on to a weight plate, dumbbell, or kettlebell for added resistance. The weighted crunch is performed in the same manner as a regular crunch (page 92), except the arms are extended above your chest to hold a weight at full arm's length.

1 Lie flat on your back on the floor with your knees bent and feet flat on the floor. With the weight in hand, extend your arms above your chest to hold the weight at full arm's length.

2 To perform the repetition, press your lower back into the floor and raise your shoulders, pushing the weight toward the ceiling, and then return to the starting position.

Leg Raise to Hip Thrust

3 SETS 12 to 15 reps each

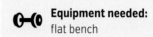

Equipment needed:
flat bench

You may choose to perform the leg raise to hip thrust or the reverse crunch, opposite. The leg raise to hip thrust works the lower portion of the abdominal muscles while raising the legs to 90 degrees and then raising the hips to push the feet toward the ceiling.

1 Lie on the bench and grasp the sides of it near your head.

2 With legs fully extended, raise your legs 90 degrees while keeping your knees locked.

3 At 90 degrees, push your feet toward the ceiling and raise your hips several inches (10 to 15 cm) off the bench to engage your lower ab muscles.

4 Lower your hips to the bench while keeping your legs straight up toward the ceiling to complete the repetition.

5 Keep your knees locked and lower your legs from the 90-degree position back to fully extended and parallel with the bench.

Reverse Crunch

3 SETS

12 to 15 reps each

Equipment needed:
flat bench

Instead of the leg raise to hip thrust, opposite, you may choose to perform the reverse crunch, which works the lower portion of the abdominal muscles while bringing the knees toward the chest to roll the hips upward.

1 Lie on the bench and grasp the sides of it near your head.

2 With legs fully extended, draw your knees toward your chest and allow your hips to roll up off the bench to engage your lower abdominal muscles.

3 Push your feet forward to a fully extended leg position to complete the repetition.

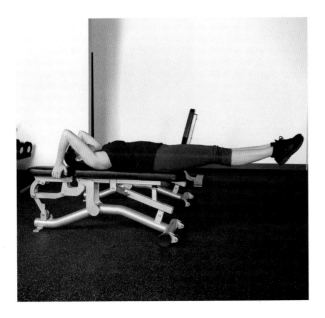

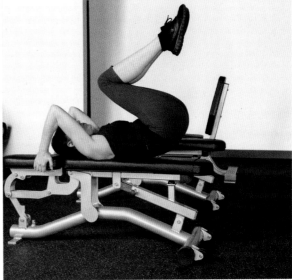

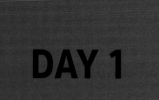

DAY 1

CHEST, TRICEPS, AND ABS

In Weeks 2 and 4 of Phase 2, we will follow the same pattern of muscles being worked as in Weeks 1 and 3, but we will change the exercises to provide more variety in the workout. For example, Day 1 will still work the same muscles (chest, triceps, and abdominals), but it will feature different exercises or variations.

On Day 1, we are working the chest, triceps, and abdominal muscles. Triceps are grouped with the chest because they are the secondary muscle used in all chest movements. People who experience symptoms of fatigue or overheating should be particularly careful when training in this phase. Use of a spotter, whenever possible, is always recommended.

Incline Bench Press

3 SETS ▶ 12 to 15 reps each   **⊶** **Equipment needed:** incline bench with dumbbells or Smith machine with bar (with or without weight plates)

This exercise works the muscles of the chest with an emphasis on the upper chest. It also works the shoulders and triceps while lifting either a bar (supported by the Smith Machine) or dumbbells over the chest. You have a choice of which equipment you use and can alternate these as you desire.

1 If using an adjustable bench, set the incline at approximately 30 degrees, which is the optimal angle to work the upper chest.

2 Grip the bar or dumbbells with a slightly wider-than-shoulder-width grip. The starting position should be across your upper chest.

3 Squeeze the muscles of your chest as you press the weight over your chest. If using dumbbells, bring the dumbbells together over your chest as you press upward.

4 With controlled movement, return the weight to the starting position to complete the repetition. Avoid letting the weight fall back to the starting position or bouncing off your chest to begin the next rep because this can cause injury.

Smith Machine Incline Bench Press

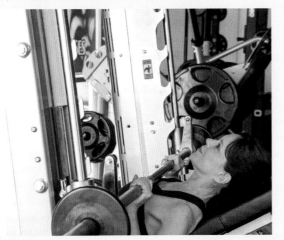 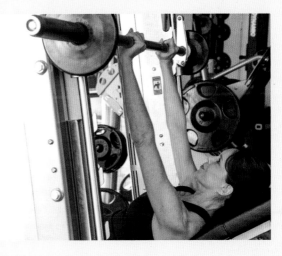

Incline Bench Press with Dumbbells

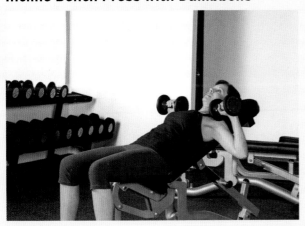 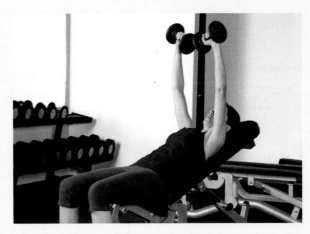

Dumbbell Fly

3 SETS   15 to 20 reps each

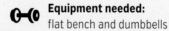 **Equipment needed:**
flat bench and dumbbells

This exercise works the chest muscles, with an emphasis on the outer chest during the stretch position and the inner chest during the contracted position, as well as the shoulders, while starting in a wide, arms outstretched position and moving to a contracted position in front of the body.

1 Lie on the bench. Starting with a dumbbell in each hand, arms outstretched above your chest, and elbows slightly bent, lower the weight in an arcing motion until your hands are aligned with your shoulders, and your elbows are slightly below chest level to stretch your chest muscles.

2 Squeeze your chest muscles and then return the dumbbells to the starting position in a reverse arcing motion. Keep a slight bend in your elbows to avoid overextending your shoulder.

3 Also, keep the bend in your elbows at a minimum to avoid engaging your biceps muscles in the movement.

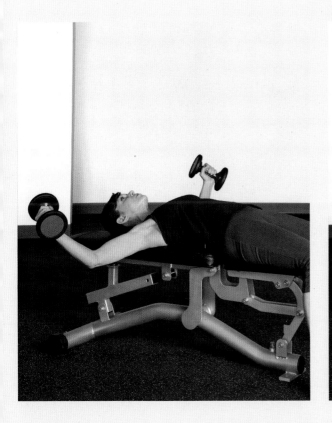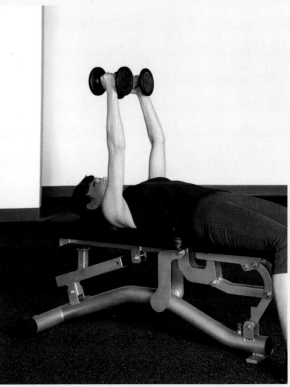

Cable Crossover or Incline Pec Deck Fly

3 SETS — 15 to 20 reps each

 Equipment needed:
cable crossover machine or pec deck machine

The cable crossover works the chest muscles, with an emphasis on the outer chest during the stretch position and the inner chest during the contracted position, as well as the shoulders, while starting in a wide, arms outstretched position and moving to a contracted position in front of the body.

The incline pec deck fly works the chest and shoulder muscles in the same way as the cable crossover while gripping the handles of the pec deck machine with a slightly higher grip and leaning slightly forward to create an incline angle. The upper portion of the chest will be worked primarily due to the incline angle. You have a choice of equipment and can alternate these, as you desire.

1 Sit with your hips against the seat back and your back arched so your shoulders are forward and in front of the pad, not in contact with it.

2 Starting with your arms outstretched to your side and elbows slightly bent, contract your chest muscles as you bring the weight forward in an arcing motion until your hands come together in front of your chest.

3 Squeeze your chest muscles and then return the handles to the starting position in a reverse arcing motion, keeping a slight bend in your elbows to avoid overextending your shoulder.

4 Also, keep the bend in your elbows at a minimum to avoid engaging your biceps muscles in the movement.

Cable Crossover

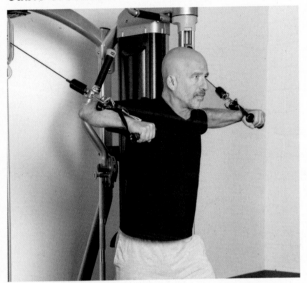 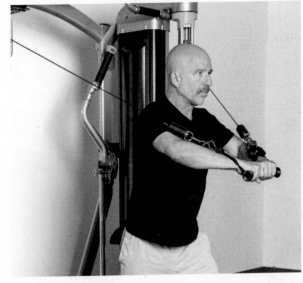

Incline Pec Deck Fly

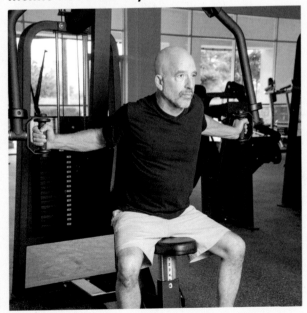 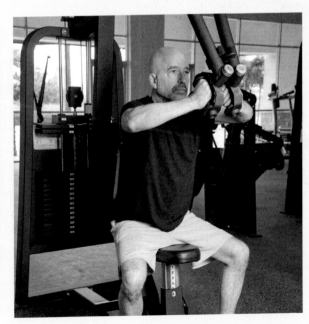

Lying Triceps Extension or Cable Lying Triceps Extension

3 SETS   12 to 15 reps each

Equipment needed: flat bench, bar of your choice, or cable machine with pulley, and bar attachment

The lying triceps extension works the triceps muscles while lying flat on a bench holding a bar or barbell over the chest and bending at the elbows to lower the weight toward the head.

The cable lying triceps extension is performed in the same manner as the lying triceps extension except a straight bar attachment or E-Z curl bar attachment is attached to a low pulley machine.

1 While lying on the bench, grasp the bar attachment of a low pulley machine.

2 From a starting position with your elbows upright and perpendicular to your body, bend at your elbow and lower your hands to bring the weight to your forehead or slightly behind your head, keeping your elbows upright and perpendicular to your body.

3 Contract your triceps muscles and raise the weight to the starting position. Keep your upper arm stationary and moving only from the elbow like a hinge, to complete the repetition.

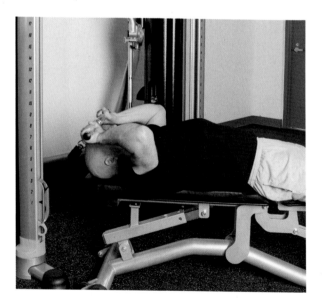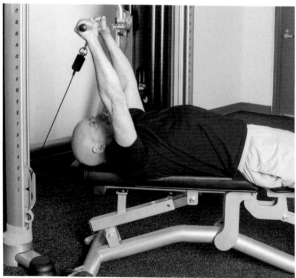

Overhead Triceps Extension

3 SETS

15 to 20 reps each

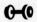 **Equipment needed:** bench, dumbbell, or cable machine with pulley in the low position, rope attachment

The overhead triceps extension exercise works the triceps muscles while raising a dumbbell overhead or by using a cable machine to work the triceps muscles while standing with your back to a cable machine and raising the weight overhead using a rope attachment connected to a low pulley.

1 From a seated position on the bench with your arms extended overhead, grasp a dumbbell with both hands around the upper weight while allowing the weight to hang.

2 Lower the weight behind your head by bending your elbows to a position of slightly less than 90 degrees.

3 Flex your triceps muscles and extend the weight to an overhead, locked-out position to complete the repetition.

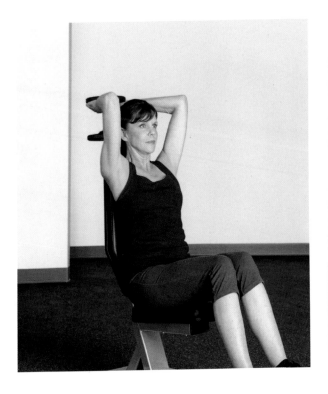

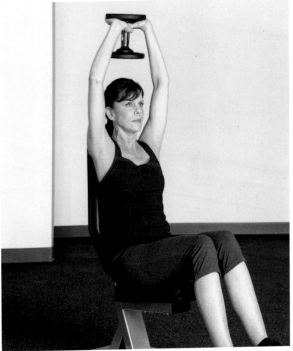

Triceps Pushdown

3 SETS 12 to 15 reps each

Equipment needed: cable machine with pulley in the high position and straight bar or V-bar attachment

This exercise, using a high pulley cable machine, works the triceps muscles while keeping the elbows near the ribs and extending the arms in front of the body to a fully extended position.

1 Stand with your knees slightly bent and feet together, or one foot slightly forward for balance. Grip the bar and keep your elbows on your ribs, close to your body.

2 Moving your arm from the elbow like a hinge, squeeze the triceps muscles and press the weight downward to a fully extended position.

3 To complete the repetition, keep your elbows at your ribs and return the weight to the starting position with your hands ending at chest level.

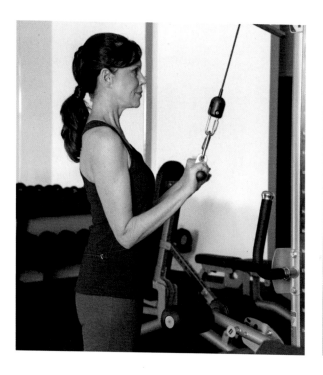 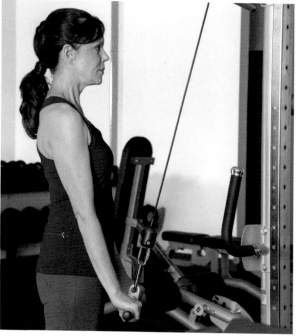

Weighted Sit-Ups

3 SETS | 20 to 25 reps each

Equipment needed:
weight plate, dumbbell, or kettlebell

This exercise works the abdominal muscles while holding a weight plate, dumbbell, or kettlebell for added resistance and raising the body to a fully seated position.

1 The weighted sit-up is performed in the same manner as a regular sit-up except your arms are extended to hold a weight a full arm's length above your head. Your feet should be placed flat on the floor with your knees bent.

2 To perform the repetition, press your lower back into the floor and roll your shoulders forward while simultaneously bringing the weight to a position in front of your feet and then return to the starting position.

Medicine Ball Russian Twist

3 SETS | 25 to 50 reps each

Equipment needed:
medicine ball

This exercise works the abdominal and oblique muscles while moving a medicine ball from side to side across the body in a rotational movement.

1 Sit on the floor with your knees slightly bent and feet out in front, heels resting lightly on the floor or slightly off the floor for added difficulty, and upper body angled back about 45 degrees. Grasp a medicine ball in front of your abdominal muscles.

2 To perform the repetition, rotate your upper body and touch the medicine ball to the floor on one side of your body while keeping your legs in a stationary position.

3 Bring the medicine ball across your body and touch the floor on the opposite side of your body. Turn your head, not just your shoulders, and look at the ball to rotate the entire midsection.

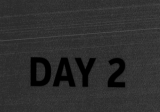
SHOULDERS, LEGS, AND CALVES

In Day 2 of Phase 2, the shoulder, leg, and calf muscles are worked. This day contains some more advanced compound movements, so anyone who experiences symptoms of fatigue or spasticity in the arms should be careful when pressing the weight overhead. Anyone with lower back issues should be very careful when performing movements that load weight onto the spine and should consider using a lifting belt if attempting these movements. As always, we recommend the use of a spotter whenever possible.

Dumbbell Lateral Raise

3 SETS ▶ 12 to 15 reps each

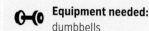 **Equipment needed:** dumbbells

This exercise works the muscles of the shoulders with an emphasis on the medial head while raising the dumbbells to the sides of the body.

1 Start with the dumbbells at your sides or in front of your body with your palms facing inward and a slight bend in your elbows.

2 Keeping the bend in your elbows consistent, lift the dumbbells straight out to your sides and away from your body to a position parallel to the floor.

3 Return the dumbbells to the starting position in a controlled movement to complete the repetition. Avoid swinging the weights to prevent injury.

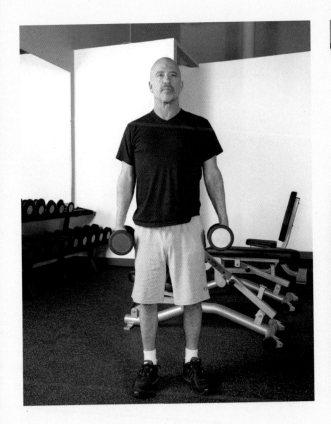
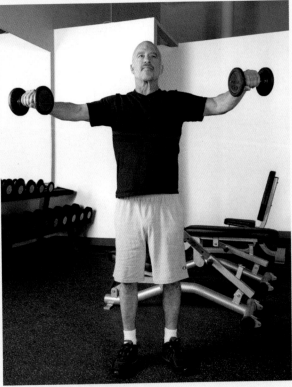

Cable Front Raise

3 SETS   12 to 15 reps each

 Equipment needed: cable machine with pulley in the low position, 2 long handles or straight bar attachment

You have the option to perform the cable front raise or dumbbell front raise, opposite. The cable front raise works the shoulder muscles, with an emphasis on the anterior head, while facing a cable machine and raising the handles to an overhead position.

1 With a straight bar attachment on a low pulley machine, take a stance with your feet slightly wider than shoulder width and your knees slightly bent, abs tight.

2 With your arms fully extended to grasp the weight in front of your body, raise your arms to an overhead position while only moving at the shoulder joint.

3 With controlled movement, lower the weight to the starting position to complete the repetition.

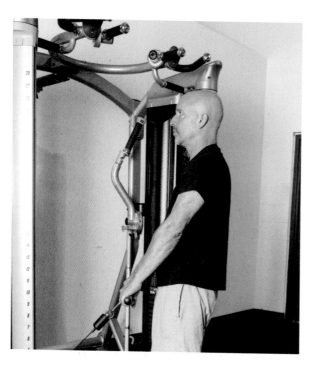 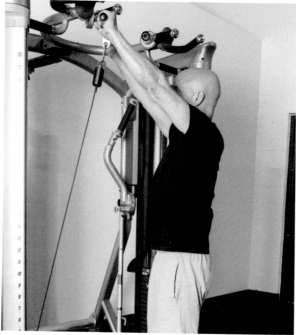

Dumbbell Front Raise

3 SETS

12 to 15 reps each

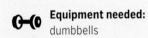

Equipment needed:
dumbbells

Instead of the cable front raise, opposite, you can perform the dumbbell front raise. This exercise works the shoulder muscles, with an emphasis on the anterior head, while raising the dumbbells to the front of the body.

1 Start with the dumbbells in front of your body with your palms resting on your thighs and your elbows slightly bent to avoid stress on your joints.

2 Lift the dumbbells straight up in front of your body to eye level. This can be done simultaneously, or alternating.

3 With controlled movement, return the dumbbells to the starting position to complete the repetition. Avoid swinging the weights to prevent injury.

Bent-Over Dumbbell Lateral Raise

3 SETS 12 to 15 reps each

 Equipment needed:
dumbbells and flat bench (optional)

This exercise works the shoulder muscles, with an emphasis on the posterior head, while raising the dumbbells out to the sides of the body in a bent-over position with the upper body parallel to the floor. You can perform this exercise either in a standing or seated position.

1 Stand with your feet together and knees slightly bent. Keep your lower back tucked in to prevent injury and bend forward until your upper body is parallel to the floor.

2 Start with the dumbbells in front of your body, under your chest, with palms facing each other and elbows slightly bent. If seated, sit on the edge of the bench and lean forward with your chest on your thighs. Start with the dumbbells underneath your legs and palms facing together.

3 Keeping your upper body parallel to the floor and your elbows slightly bent, raise the dumbbells to the outside in an arcing motion. Keep your shoulders, elbows, and hands all in the same plane of movement.

4 With controlled movement, return the dumbbells to the starting position to complete the repetition.

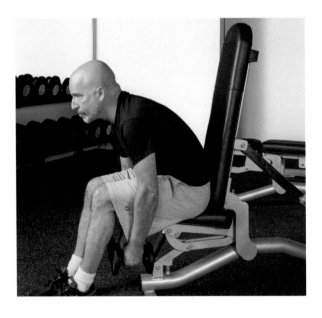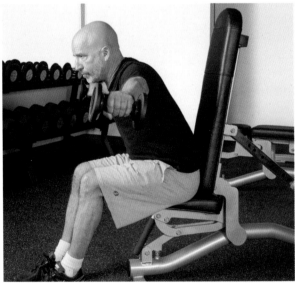

Leg Press

4 SETS

15 to 20 reps each

Equipment needed:
leg press machine

This exercise works the quadriceps, hamstrings, and gluteal muscles while seated in a leg press machine and pressing the weight upward at a 45-degree angle.

1 Sit in the leg press machine with your back firmly against the pad and your feet on the plate about shoulder width apart. Release the safety handles to lower the weight.

2 With controlled movement, lower the weight by bending at your knees and hips, bringing your thighs toward your chest, and keeping your knees aligned with your toes.

3 To complete the repetition, contract the quadriceps muscles and press the weight back to the starting position.

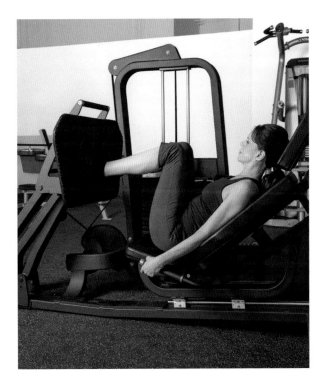

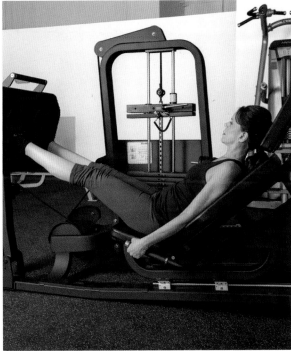

Leg Extension

3 SETS 15 to 20 reps each

Equipment needed:
leg extension machine

This exercise works the quadriceps muscles while sitting in a leg extension machine and extending the legs in front of the body.

1 Sit in the machine with your back placed firmly against the back pad and the lower pad on the front of your ankle. Your knee joint should be in alignment with the machine's pivot point.

2 Simultaneously raise your legs to their full extension.

3 Squeeze your quadriceps muscles at the top of the movement before lowering the weight, with controlled movement, back to the starting position to complete the repetition.

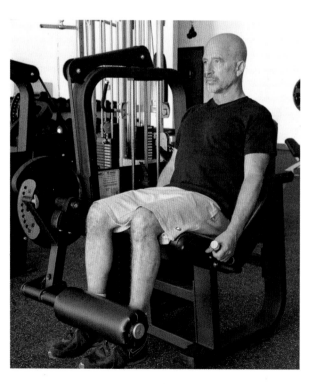

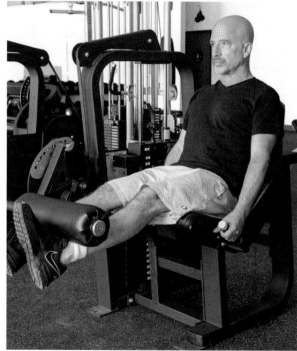

Seated Leg Curl

3 SETS   15 to 20 reps each

Equipment needed: seated leg curl machine

This exercise works the hamstring muscles while seated in a leg curl machine with the legs extended in front of the body and curling the weight under the seat.

1 Sit in the machine with your back pressed firmly against the pad. Your feet will be straight in front with the pad behind your ankles. Your knee joint should be in alignment with the machine's pivot point.

2 To perform the repetition, contract your hamstring muscles and lower the weight, with controlled movement, to a position under the seat.

3 With controlled movement, return the weight to the starting position to complete the repetition.

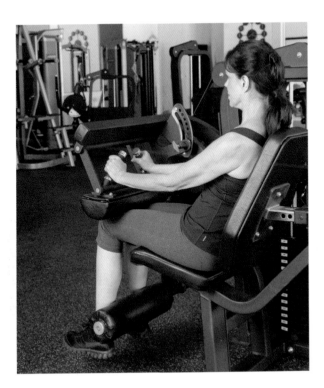

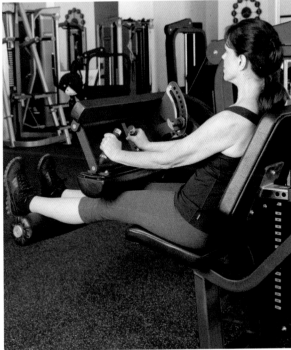

Stiff Leg Dead Lift

3 SETS 15 to 20 reps each

Equipment needed: fixed-weight barbell or bar (with or without weight plates)

This exercise works the hamstring muscles and the gluteal muscles while holding a barbell or bar in front of the body and pushing the hips backward to lower it toward the floor while avoiding bending at the knees.

1 Start from an upright position with your feet 6 to 8 in (15 to 20 cm) apart and your lower back tucked in to avoid injury. You knees should be unlocked and your legs just slightly bent in a "stiff" but not "straight" position.

2 Push your hips backward and bring your shoulders down. Keep your shoulders pulled back and back flat while hanging the barbell or bar at arm's length and close to your body.

3 To complete the repetition, contract your upper leg muscles (gluteals and hamstrings) and return to an upright position.

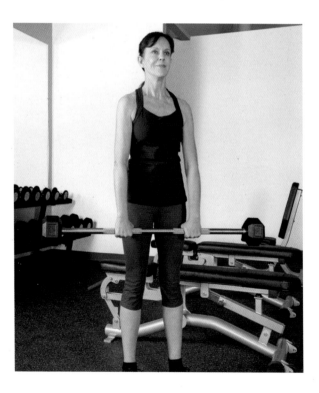

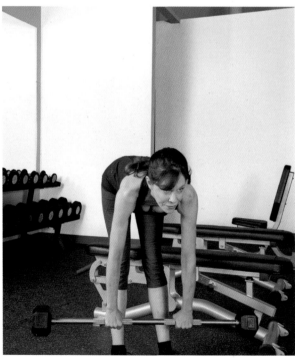

Leg Press Calf Raise

3 SETS

20 to 25 reps each

Equipment needed:
leg press machine

This exercise works the calf muscles, with an emphasis on the gastrocnemius muscle, while supporting the sled of a leg press machine on the balls of the feet and extending the ankles.

1 Sit in the leg press machine and place the balls of your feet on the platform.

2 Keeping your knees in an unlocked position, press the weight by pushing up on your toes until your calf muscles are fully contracted.

3 To complete the repetition, lower the weight to a point where your heels are below your toes to a fully stretched position of the calf muscles.

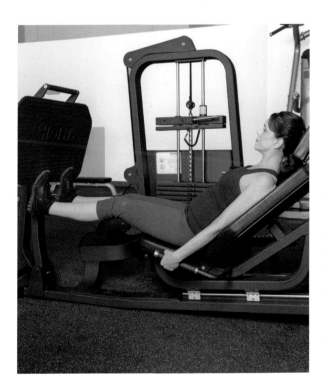
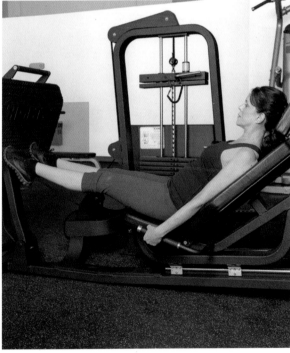

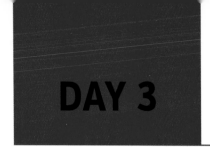

DAY 3

BACK, BICEPS, AND ABS

On Day 3 of Phase 2, we are working the back, biceps, and abdominal muscles. Biceps are grouped with the back because they are the secondary muscle used in all back movements. People who experience symptoms of fatigue or neuropathy in the hands should be extremely careful when gripping a weight in an overhead position. As always, the use of a spotter is recommended for safety, when possible.

Pull-Ups or Assisted Pull-Ups

4 SETS — 12 to 15 reps each

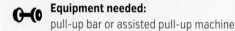 **Equipment needed:**
pull-up bar or assisted pull-up machine

Pull-ups are one of the best exercises to work the back muscles, with an emphasis on the lats. They also work the shoulder and biceps muscles while starting from a full hang position and pulling the body upward.

The assisted pull-up is performed while kneeling on an assisted pull-up machine in a full hang position and pulling the body upward, allowing the machine to assist with a portion of the body weight.

1 Grasp a pull-up bar with a wide grip and hang at a full arm's length.

2 To perform the repetition, pull your body up to a position where your chin is above the bar, keeping your back arched and chest up.

3 With controlled movement, lower your body so that it's fully extended and at the starting position to complete the repetition.

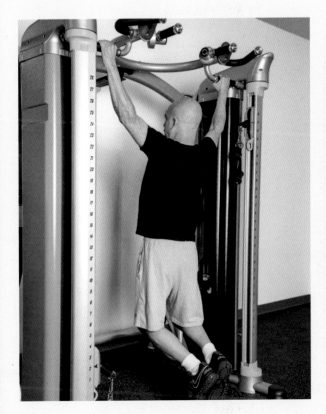 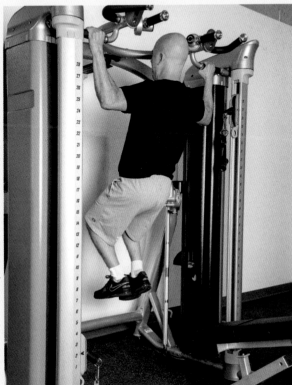

Two-Hand Dumbbell Row

3 SETS — 15 to 20 reps each

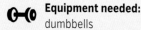 **Equipment needed:** dumbbells

This exercise works the mid-back muscles, with an emphasis on the rhomboids and lats, as well as the shoulders and biceps, while holding two dumbbells in front of the body in a slightly bent-over position and pulling the dumbbells toward the ribs on the side of the body.

1 With your feet together, bend at your waist to a position where your chest is almost parallel to the floor while holding a dumbbell in each hand.

2 With your arms fully extended and the dumbbells hanging toward the floor, row the dumbbells upward, toward your ribs while simultaneously pushing your elbows toward the ceiling, chest toward the floor, and squeezing your shoulder blades together.

3 With controlled movement, lower the weight to a fully extended position and relax your shoulder blades to complete the repetition.

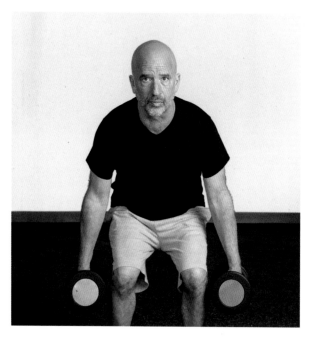
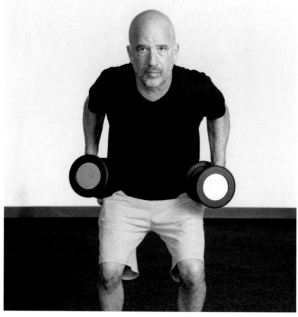

Reverse-Grip Lat Pulldown

3 SETS

15 to 20 reps each

Equipment needed:
lat pulldown machine and lat bar attachment

This exercise works the back muscles, with an emphasis on the lats, rhomboids, shoulders, and biceps, while pulling a weight from overhead toward the upper chest with a grip on the bar with the palms facing toward the body.

1 While sitting in a lat pulldown machine, grasp the bar with a reverse grip, hands approximately 12 in (30 cm) apart with your palms facing toward your body.

2 Pull the weight toward your collarbone while simultaneously pushing your chest up toward the bar and squeezing your shoulder blades together.

3 Relax your shoulder blades and extend the weight overhead to a full arm's length to complete the repetition.

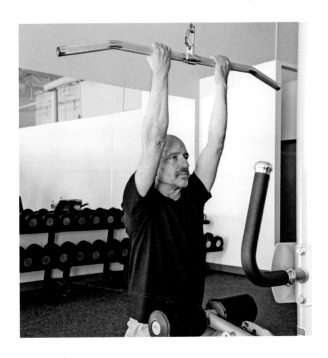

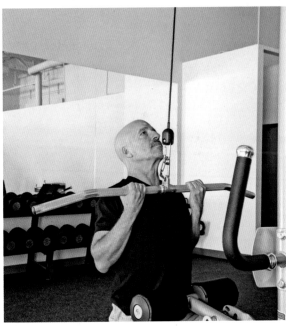

Incline Dumbbell Curl

3 SETS ▶ 12 to 15 reps each

Equipment needed:
incline or adjustable bench and dumbbells

This exercise works the biceps muscles, with an emphasis on the long head of the muscle, while seated on an inclined bench and curling the weight from a hanging position upward toward the shoulders.

1 Sit in an adjustable bench with the angle set at around 45 degrees. Begin with a dumbbell in each hand and let your arms hang at your sides, palms facing forward.

2 Squeeze your biceps and curl the weight up toward your shoulders.

3 With controlled movement, lower the weight back to the starting position to complete the repetition.

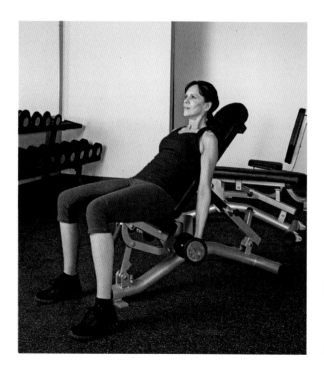
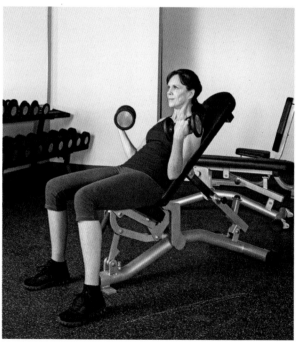

High Cable Curl

3 SETS

15 to 20 reps each

Equipment needed: high pulley machine and straight bar attachment

This exercise works the biceps muscles using a high pulley machine with straight bar attachment and curling the weight toward the forehead.

1 Stand in front of a high pulley machine and grasp a straight bar attachment with your arms extended in front of your body.

2 Keeping your elbows stationary in front of your body, contract your biceps and curl the weight toward your forehead.

3 Continue to keep your elbows stationary in front of the body and relax your biceps, allowing the weight to move forward to a full arm's length to complete the repetition.

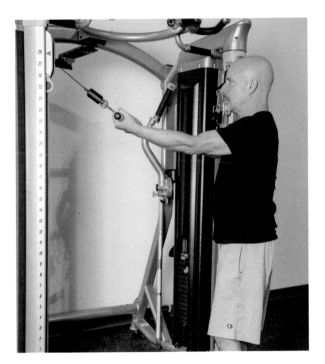
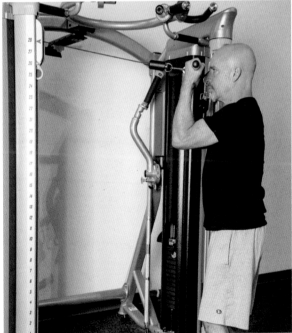

Rope Hammer Curl

3 SETS 15 to 20 reps each

Equipment needed: cable machine with pulley in the low position and rope attachment

For this exercise, you may choose to perform the rope hammer curl or preacher curl (page 120). The rope hammer curl works the biceps muscles, with an emphasis on the short head of the muscle, as well as the brachialis muscle, while curling a weight up toward the shoulders with a rope attachment connected to a low pulley.

1 Stand facing the cable machine, keeping your knees unlocked and core muscles tight. Grasp the rope with a thumbs-up grip and your elbows slightly in front of your body.

2 To perform the repetition, squeeze your biceps and curl the weight up toward your shoulders while keeping the thumbs-up hand position and elbows in front of your body.

3 With controlled movement, lower the weight to the starting position to complete the repetition. Avoid swinging the weight to prevent lower back injuries.

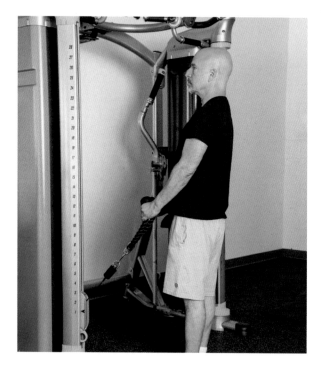
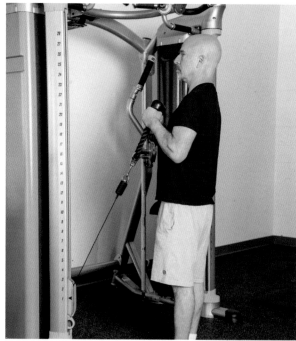

Weighted Sit-Ups

3 SETS ▶ 20 to 25 reps each

Equipment needed:
weight plate, dumbbell, or kettlebell

This exercise works the abdominal muscles while holding a weight plate, dumbbell, or kettlebell for added resistance and raising the body to a fully seated position.

1 The weighted sit-up is performed in the same manner as a regular sit-up except your arms are extended to hold a weight a full arm's length above your head. Your feet should be placed flat on the floor with your knees bent.

2 To perform the repetition, press your lower back into the floor and roll your shoulders forward while simultaneously bringing the weight to a position in front of your feet and then return to the starting position.

Medicine Ball Russian Twist

 3 SETS 25 to 50 reps each

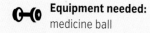 **Equipment needed:**
medicine ball

This exercise works the abdominal and oblique muscles while moving a medicine ball from side to side across the body in a rotational movement.

1 Sit on the floor with your knees slightly bent and feet out in front, heels resting lightly on the floor or slightly off the floor for added difficulty, and upper body angled back approximately 45 degrees. Grasp a medicine ball in front of your abdomin.

2 To perform the repetition, rotate your upper body and touch the medicine ball to the floor on one side of your body while keeping your legs in a stationary position.

3 Bring the medicine ball across your body and touch the floor on the opposite side of your body. Turn your head, not just your shoulders, and look at the ball to rotate your entire midsection.

 Note

- If you are training for more than three days, repeat the workouts in sequence.

- Metabolism jump-start exercises do not replace your regular cardio session. They are only meant to burn additional calories during your workout.

- If time allows, do an additional thirty minutes of steady cardio immediately following your workout.

WHAT NOW?

You've completed both phases of the OptimalBody HD Training System. By now, you should have enough exercises in your fitness arsenal and enough experience and confidence to create some killer workouts. You can also use the workouts from the different phases in different order to stimulate your muscles in different ways. For example, you could begin again with a Phase 2 workout and alternate with a Phase 1 workout, or simply start again with Phase 1. It's always a good idea to return to the basics every now and then and revisit the strength building routines of Phase 1. You'll probably be surprised at how much stronger you have gotten since beginning Phase 1 of your journey. The possibilities are endless, and as long as you don't get stuck in a routine, your muscles will continue to respond.

At OptimalBody, we believe that a strong mind and a strong body are the two most important things a person can possess. Know that you can accomplish anything!

No matter what types of limitations you face, remember they are simply limitations, not a reason to give up on your goals. We all deserve to live life to the fullest, and, while that may differ from person to person, we each are in control of what that means to us. We can take what is handed to us and accept it as all that we will have, or we can rise up to face adversity and create a life of value where we continually strive to push the limits of what we are capable of. At OptimalBody, we believe that a strong mind and a strong body are the two most important things a person can possess. Know that you can accomplish anything!

ACKNOWLEDGMENTS

So many people and companies have supported my decision to take this journey into fitness with multiple sclerosis. It would take me a book to thank them all, but I must acknowledge a few here.

Many thanks go to my literary agent, Marilyn Allen, who heard my story and felt my passion to share my knowledge so I can encourage and educate those people who need it the most, and to my editor, Brunella Costagliola, who endured my constant pestering along the way. Patience is her middle name! Thank you to Jess Haberman and everyone at Fair Winds Press who had the confidence in me to publish this book.

I am grateful to be in the company of amazing and genuine people, such as personal trainer and fitness director for my MS Fitness Challenge charity, Darren Barnes, who helped get me out of my house and into the gym to start this journey; long-time friend Michael Torchia, former bodybuilding champion and current celebrity fitness trainer, who has been behind me along the way; IFBB pro bodybuilder and contest prep coach Chris Williamson, who is always there for me as I try to perfect my imperfect body; and Arnold Schwarzenegger, who made a dream come true when he handed me the Health Advocate Lifetime Achievement Award at the Arnold Classic sports event in March 2015.

Thank you to Randall McClain, D.O., my sports medicine doctor who monitors my health like a hawk. He has told me, from our first visit, that I should keep pushing forward as a hardcore bodybuilder, to do what makes me happy, and that he has my back. He certainly does, as a doctor and a friend.

Thanks to my business partner at Bishop-Lyons Entertainment, Andrew Bishop, who allows me to pursue my dreams in fitness and build my charity to help others with MS do the same. He tows the line so I can battle MS on my battlefield.

Thanks to the Global Bodybuilding Organization, which has acknowledged me at its fitness events nationwide and honored me with the Lifetime Fitness Inspiration Award in February 2016; nutritional supplement company Champion Performance, which has sponsored my MS cause and my bodybuilding in a major way; and all the trainers, participants, and supporters of the MS Fitness Challenge charity and our director of trainers, Mark Mueller, who proves the way to battle this disease is through fitness and nutrition.

I am humbled by their encouragement and thankful for each and every one of my supporters.

As I thank as many of my supporters as possible I can never forget my friend Luke Wood, six-time winner of the Australian Bodybuilding Championships and one of the greatest bodybuilders to ever step on stage. Luke reached out to me from across the world in Australia when he heard I was bodybuilding with MS to lend his advice and more importantly his encouragement. Sadly Luke died at the age of 35 in 2011 from complications stemming from a kidney transplant. He is tremendously missed. R.I.P. Big Luke.

SUPPORTERS AND ENDORSERS

Many people and companies have supported, endorsed, and/or been a part of my efforts to positively impact the lives of those with MS and other chronic conditions. These are my current supporters/endorsers.

American CryoStem Corporation
www.americancryostem.com

American Fitness Professionals & Associates
http://store.afpafitness.com/ms-fitness-wellness-specialist-1

Arnold (Schwarzenegger) Fitness Expo
www.arnoldsportsfestival.com/splash

BioTrust Nutrition
http://msfitness.biotrust.com

Bishop Lyons Entertainment
www.bishoplyons.com

Bodybuilding.com
www.bodybuilding.com/fun/lyons-roar-bodybuilder-battles-multiple-sclerosis.html

Champion Performance
www.championperformance.com

Climb New Heights
www.climbnewheights.com

Daymond John
http://daymondjohn.com

Egg Crystals
www.eggcrystals.com

Everyday Health
www.everydayhealth.com/columns/ms-fitness-challenge

Fellowship of Christian Athletes
www.fca.org

Global Bodybuilding Organization
www.globalbodybuildingorganization.com

Goldy Locks
www.goldylocksband.com

Jackie's Groove
entertalkradio.com/jackiesgroove

Legion Athletics
https://legionathletics.com

Medical Fitness Network
https://medicalfitnessnetwork.org

Michael Torchia's Elite Health Concierge Service
operationfitness.com

Multiple Sclerosis Foundation
www.msfocus.com

OptimalBody Personal Fitness
optimalbodypersonalfitness.com

Polar Products
www.polarproducts.com/polarshop/pc/home.asp

Ric Drasin/Ric's Corner
www.youtube.com/watch?v=bNI96XoPTjw

Tony Little
www.tonylittle.com

WEGO Health
www.wegohealth.com

ABOUT THE AUTHORS

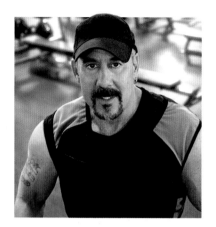

David Lyons was a healthy bodybuilder and gym owner when he was diagnosed with MS in 2006 at the age of forty-seven. The doctors told him he would rapidly decline and require a wheelchair. Instead David battled the disease in the gym and challenged himself by competing in an NPC bodybuilding competition. David and his wife, Kendra, then founded the MS Fitness Challenge, which provides certified fitness professionals to people with MS nationwide for twelve weeks at no cost, as well as a gym membership, in an effort to educate and train them in the benefits of exercise and nutrition. He and Kendra have also launched their own gym, the Optimal-Body Personal Fitness facility, in Murrieta, CA.

With American Fitness Professionals & Associates (AFPA), David developed the MS Fitness & Wellness Specialist certification. He currently writes for EverydayHealth.com. David was the recipient of the Most Inspirational Award at the 2009 Florida State Bodybuilding Championship at fifty years old, the National MS Society Milestone Award, the Health Advocate Achievement Award (alongside Lou Ferrigno), the Health Advocate Lifetime Achievement Award (presented by Arnold Schwarzenegger), and the Lifetime Fitness Inspiration Award from the Global Bodybuilding Organization.

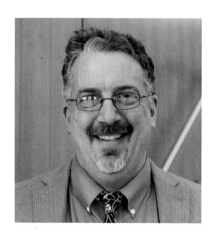

Jacob Sloane, M.D., Ph.D., is a neurologist at the multiple sclerosis clinic at Beth Israel Deaconess Medical Center in Boston, working to enhance the high-level care of MS patients at this institution and to conduct multiple sclerosis–related research. He is a graduate of Harvard University and Boston University Medical School. His Ph.D. in pathology was performed in Carmela Abraham's laboratory at Boston University. He completed an internship at Beth Israel Deaconess Medical Center and a neurology residency at Massachusetts General Hospital and Brigham and Women's Hospital. He started his own laboratory in 2009.

APPENDIX

Sample Fitness and Nutrition Journal

Goals

_____

_____

_____

_____

Diet and Nutrition

	Calories	Protein	Fiber	Carbs	Fat	Comments
Breakfast: _____						
Lunch: _____						
Dinner: _____						
Snacks and beverages: _____						

Exercise

Exercise	Set 1: lb (kg)	Set 1: reps	Set 2: lb (kg)	Set 2: reps	Set 3: lb (kg)	Set 3: reps

INDEX

A

Adaptations, workout, 54, 55, 57–58, 60–66. *See also* Wheelchair adaptations
Air squat (body weight squat), 122
Alternating body weight lunges, 123
Anti-inflammatory diet, 32, 33–44, 45, 46
Anti-inflammatory lifestyle, 44–45

B

Back, biceps, and abs exercises
    Phase 1, Day 3
        barbell curl, 116–17
        barbell row, 114
        incline dumbbell curl, 118
        preacher curl, 120
        pull-ups or assisted pull-ups, 108–9
        rope hammer curl, 119
        seated cable row, 110–11
        straight-arm lat pulldown, 115
        wide-grip lat pulldown, 112–13
    Phase 2, Day 3
        barbell curl, 150
        barbell row, 146–47
        cable crunch, 152
        high cable curl, 181
        incline dumbbell curl, 180
        leg raise to hip thrust, 154
        medicine ball Russian twist, 184
        preacher curl with dumbbells, 151
        pull-ups or assisted pull-ups, 176–77
        reverse crunch, 155
        reverse-grip lat pulldown, 179
        rope hammer curl, 182
        seated cable row, 149
        two-hand dumbbell row, 178
        weighted crunch, 153
        weighted sit-ups, 183
        wide-grip lat pulldown, 148
Balance problems, adaptations for, 65
Beverages, 39, 42, 43
Bodybuilding, as motivation, 12–16
Burnout, 29

C

Cardiovascular training, 59, 66, 69
Chest, shoulders, triceps, and abs exercises (Phase 1, Day 1)
    bent-over dumbbell lateral raise, 80–81
    crunch, 92
    dumbbell front raise, 79
    dumbbell lateral raise, 78
    dumbbell shoulder press, 76–77
    hip thrust, 91
    incline bench press, 70–71
    incline dumbbell fly or cable crossover, 74–75
    knee tuck, 90
    leg raise, 88–89
    lying triceps extension, 82
    machine chest press, 72–73
    medicine ball Russian twist, 93
    overhead cable triceps extension, 86–87
    triceps dip, 83
    triceps pushdown, 84–85
Chest, triceps, and abs exercises (Phase 2, Day 1)
    bench dip, 128
    cable crossover or incline pec deck fly, 160–61
    cable crunch, 130
    chest press, 124–25
    close-grip bench press, 129
    dumbbell fly, 158–59
    incline bench press, 156–57
    incline bench press with dumbbells, 126
    leg raise to hip thrust, 132
    lying triceps extension or cable lying triceps extension, 162
    medicine ball Russian twist, 165
    overhead triceps extension, 163
    pec deck fly, 127
    reverse crunch, 133
    triceps pushdown, 164
    weighted crunch, 131
    weighted sit-ups, 165
Circuit training, 60, 61, 67
Coconut palm sugar, 43

D

Dairy foods, anti-inflammatory, 38
Diet. *See* Nutrition
Doctors, communicating with, 22
Doctor's Notes, 9
    communication with doctors, 22
    diet, 21, 31, 32, 33, 34, 51
    exercise, 18, 20, 21, 22, 55, 59
    fatigue and exercise, 15, 57
    heat sensitivity, 20
    inflammation, 31
    injuries, 13, 21
    meditation, 24
    osteopenia and osteoporosis, 58
    overweight, 59
    sugar, 42
    yoga, 25

E

Exercise(s). *See also specific exercises*
    as anti-inflammatory, 44
    eating guidelines for, 47–48
    modifying, 61–62

F

Faith, inspiration from, 17
Fatigue, as MS symptom, 15, 19, 29, 55
    circuit training and, 60
    diet and, 32, 34, 42, 47, 51
    exercise safety with, 21, 57, 70, 124,
      134, 146, 156, 166, 176
    injuries from, 13, 21
    reducing, 24, 25, 51, 59
    workout challenge from, 13,
      14, 15, 18
Fats, 38, 42
Fitness, as lifestyle, 22
Foods to avoid, 34, 42
Fruits, anti-inflammatory, 36

G

Grip impairment, adaptations for, 64–65
Gut microbiota, 31, 32

H

Heat intolerance, 13, 20, 21
Herbs, anti-inflammatory, 39
Honey, raw, 44
Hypertrophic definition (HD), 60, 68

I

Inflammation, 30–45
Injuries, 13, 14, 18, 19, 20, 21, 63, 64
Inspiration, 12, 25, 50, 51

J

Journaling, 28, 189
Jump rope, 123
Jump squat (plyometric squat), 122

L

Leg exercises (Phase 1, Day 2)
    leg extension, 94–95
    leg press, 97
    leg press calf raise, 105
    seated calf raise, 106–7
    seated leg curl, 100–101
    squat, 96
    standing calf raise, 104
    stiff leg dead lift, 102–3
    walking lunge, 98–99
Lifestyle, anti-inflammatory, 44–45
Lucuma powder, 44

M

Magnesium, 32
Meal planning, 45–46
Meditation, 23–24, 25
Mediterranean diet, 33
Medjool dates, 44
Mental challenges, 19
Mental exhaustion, 29
Mental fitness, 23
    techniques for
      exposure to nature, 28
      journaling, 28
      meditation, 23–24, 25
      positive affirmations, 25–26
      vision board, 26–28
      yoga, 24–25
Metabolism, 58
Metabolism jump-starts, 64, 121–23, 184
Mini circuits, 60
Motivation, 12–16, 22, 50, 51, 52
Mountain climber, 123
MS Bodybuilding Challenge, 16–22
Muscle building, 58–59
Muscle tears, 20, 21

N

Nature, benefits of, 28
Negative thinking, 19, 50
Numbness
    adaptations for, 64–65
    as workout challenge, 13, 15,
      18, 19, 21
Nutrition
    anti-inflammatory, 33–44, 45
    budget-friendly, 49
    healthy mind-sets for, 49–52
    meal planning and, 45–46
    MS and, 31–32
    pre- and post-workout, 47–48

O

Obesity, 32
Obstacles, 10, 55
Omega-3 fatty acids, 33
Online exercise library, 90
OptimalBody HD Training System
    aftermath of, 185
    muscles worked in, 56
    overtraining avoidance in, 64
    overview of, 10, 54–56
    phases of, 10, 54 (see also Phase 1;
      Phase 2; Phase 3)
    praise for, 8
    progressions or regressions
      in, 60–63
    purpose of, 17–18
    safety considerations in, 63,
      64–65, 66, 94
    terminology of, 57–60
    weight-lifting principles in, 20
    wheelchair adaptations in (see
      Wheelchair adaptations)
Osteopenia and osteoporosis, 58
Overtraining avoidance, 64
Overview of this book, 9–10

INDEX

P

Pain
    reducing, 25, 32, 51, 59
    as workout challenge, 13, 14, 15, 18
Phase 1, 10, 54
    adaptations in, 64–66
    Day 1 chest, shoulders, triceps, and abs exercises, 70–93
    Day 2 leg exercises, 94–107
    Day 3 back, biceps, and abs exercises, 108–20
    guidelines for, 66–69
    progressions in, 60, 61
    safety considerations in, 70, 94
Phase 2, 10, 54, 67
    Day 1 chest, triceps, and abs exercises, 124–33, 156–65
    Day 2 shoulders, legs, and calves exercises, 134–45, 166–75
    Day 3 back, biceps, and abs exercises, 146–55, 176–84
    metabolism jump-starts in, 121–23, 184
    overview of, 121
    preventing plateaus in, 64
    safety considerations in, 124, 134, 146, 156, 166, 176
Phase 3, 10, 185
Plateaus, 64
Positive affirmations, 25–26
Positive thoughts, 29, 50
Probiotic foods, 32, 38, 41
Processed foods, 42, 43, 47, 52
Progressions, in workouts, 57–58, 60, 61, 62, 63
Protein-rich foods, as anti-inflammatory, 37

R

Regressions, for modifying exercises, 54, 61, 62, 63
Repetitions (reps), 57, 58–59, 61, 64
Resistance bands, 64, 65, 66

Resistance training, 58–59
Running in place, 122

S

Sample fitness and nutrition journal, 189
Setbacks, 19–22
Sets, 57, 58–59, 63
Shoulders, legs, and calves exercises (Phase 2, Day 2)
    alternating dumbbell shoulder press, 136
    barbell shoulder press, 134–35
    bent-over dumbbell lateral raise, 170
    cable front raise, 168
    cable upright row, 139
    dead lift, 141
    dumbbell front raise, 169
    dumbbell lateral raise, 166–67
    leg extension, 172
    leg press, 171
    leg press calf raise, 144, 175
    machine shoulder press, 137
    seated calf raise, 145
    seated leg curl, 173
    Smith machine upright row, 138
    squat, 140
    standing calf raise, 143
    stiff leg dead lift, 174
    walking lunge, 142
Sleep, 45
Smith machine, 65
Smoking, 44
Spasticity
    exercise safety with, 70, 166
    magnesium reducing, 32
    as workout challenge, 13, 14, 15
Spices, anti-inflammatory, 39
Spotter
    for Phase 1, 70, 94
    for Phase 2, 124, 134, 146, 156, 166, 176
    Smith machine as, 65

Stationary lunge, modifying, 61–62
Step-ups, 122
Stevia, 43
Stress, 25, 29, 45, 54
Stretching, 68–69
Sugar and sugar alternatives, 42–44
Supersets, 60, 61
Supplements, anti-inflammatory, 32, 41
Support sources, 51–52
Sweet treats, 40
Symptoms of MS
    adaptations for, 64–65
    injuries from, 21
    workout difficulty from, 13, 14, 15, 18, 19

T

Toxin load, reducing, 44
Trainer, fitness, 15, 17, 18, 21, 22, 55, 56, 62, 63, 65
Training schedule and methods, 19–20
Training shortcuts, pitfalls of, 20

V

Vegetables, anti-inflammatory, 35
Vision board, 26–28
Vitamin D, 32

W

Warm-up, pre-workout, 69
Weight-lifting straps, 13, 18, 21, 65
Weight loss or control, 32, 45, 59
Weight selection, for sets, 63
Wheelchair adaptations, 66, 69, 72, 76, 80, 86, 91, 92, 94, 102, 106, 112, 116
Whole grains, anti-inflammatory, 36
Workout challenges with MS, 13–14, 15, 18, 19